A DOCTORS GUIDE TO CONCIERGE MEDICINE

First Edition.

*Essential Startup Steps for Doctors Considering a Career
in Concierge Medicine, DPC or Membership Medicine.*

By Michael Tetreault and Catherine Sykes

© **CONCIERGE MEDICINE TODAY, LLC**
PUBLISHER: dba "Docpreneur Press"
4080 McGinnis Ferry Road, Building 800, Suite 801, Alpharetta, Georgia 30005
www.DocPreneurPress.org | www.ConciergeMedicineToday.com

"Please do not go it alone....seek advice/guidance with those of us that have experience. Make sure you understand the medical legal aspects of this that might be very specific for your state."

~Joel Bessmer, MD, FACP, Omaha, NE

"Wise people know when they are in no condition to decide for themselves by themselves."

~Andy Stanley, Author/Pastor

In a December 2014 interview with CNN Money, a July 2014 interview with The Atlanta Journal Constitution and a May 2014 Medscape interview, Concierge Medicine Today and The DPC Journal editors report that there are nearly 4000 physicians "who are verifiably, actively practicing concierge medicine or DPC across the United States, with probably another 8000 practicing under the radar – providing the marketplace with a total of 12,000 physicians operating in either Concierge Medicine or a DPC business model in the U.S."

Free market medicine and membership medicine delivery models therefore represent approximately 1% of All Licensed Physicians In The U.S. in 2014 or 5+% of all Licensed Primary Care Physicians In The U.S. in 2014."

"Some have said, 'We're in the Golden Age of technology but Dark Ages of delivery.' We have resources but no time to utilize them to their highest & best use."
-Dr Andrea Klemes, physician and MDVIP Medical Director,
says in an interview with Medical Economics.

Dedication

To all of those visioneering doctors across America who with a stethoscope and a clear mind, come to the aid of our families and to our bedsides as friends and expert caretakers – those who truly want to "normalize" their practices and get back to practicing medicine ... like it should be done. You are pioneering a new movement in healthcare. Keep innovating!

Additionally, there are so many individuals, physicians, businesses and others who contributed to this body of work throughout the past few years. Without your proven expertise, dedication to your profession, enthusiasm for this book, and encouragement over the years, this resource would not be available. Thank you!

What Others Are Saying About Prior Books ...

Learning a lot from this book. Concierge Medicine sounds like a great way to go.
Highly suggest this book for those confused about insurance.
– Michele

Book was a very quick read. Nonetheless is a good introduction to the topic.
– Blogger

Excellent review on a subject that is really in it is infancy. Unfortunately, right now there are very
few good resources on retainer medicine and this is one of them. The author is an expert, and is also the founder and
chief editor of the website Concierge Medicine Today, currently the best and most replete resource on this topic I
have found. I am looking forward to the second,
updated edition (i.e., I am encouraging and hoping the author will write one).
– Dr. K.B., Virginia

CMT is a thought leader, resource promoter and investigative platform dedicated
to advancing Concierge Medicine throughout the medical field. They stand alone
in this mission and assist physicians in providing better care and services to their Patients.
This makes for a healthier population.
– Dr. B.T., DO, FAAP, Florida

"I met you at the conference in Costa Mesa, CA last year. I was one of the Pediatricians interested in starting my
Concierge Practice. I have since accomplished my goal. Yay!!! Your books have been a good resource for me. Thank
you for writing them, and for all the guidance that you are offering in this reviving practice. My Practice is now in
the Greater San Diego area."
– Dr. S.S, San Diego, California

What Physicians Say About Concierge Medicine ...

Source: ConciergeMedicineToday.com | www.DirectPrimaryCare.com

"I made the switch many years ago into Concierge Medicine, or at least a form of it, and I couldn't be happier. I can provide better care and build a strong relationship with my Patients. It definitely can be challenging since I make myself available 24/7, however if you can develop a good support structure of other like-minded MDs you can maintain a successful business with less stress than a traditional practice."

-Las Vegas Urgent Care Doctor

"The road was much more difficult than I expected, but also much more satisfying. I spent much of my time learning what does not work, but in the end learned that most good ideas grow out of the remains of a hundred bad ones that didn't survive."

-Rob Lamberts, MD, Augusta, GA

"I'm always ready. I make house calls. I'll go to private offices – whatever they need. I can do essentially anything that can be done in most typical doctor's offices."

-Dr. Robert Nelson, Cumming, GA

"This new practice has been truly liberating. I am working harder than ever getting it of the ground but my time with Patients is wonderful. And I get to be creative again in how I develop the practice, something that was lost from my previous office."

-Dr. Alicia Cunningham, Vermont

"I love being an old school concierge doc and look forward to helping move this to the forefront of medicine and ultimately improve the health of all Americans!."

-Dr. Ronald Primas, New York

"You will never regret being a doctor IF you work only for Patients. But if you do not work only for Patients, you will regret your decision in the end."

-Dr. Thomas LaGrelius, California

"I received a phone call today from a physician in Winter Park Florida. She was calling just to thank me for answering her questions about Concierge Medicine a few months ago, and encouraging her to start her own concierge practice. Today, her practice is thriving and she said that "she is happy with her schedule, her life, and being able to practice medicine that way it is meant to be practiced." I was so happy to hear that I helped a fellow physician and colleague, and even more happy to hear that she was doing so well! "

-Tiffany Sizemore-Ruiz, D.O., Florida

What Patients Say About Concierge Medicine ...

Source: ConciergeMedicineToday.com | www.DirectPrimaryCare.com

"Our family finally found a better way to manage healthcare and costs.
It is called Concierge Medicine."
- Jennifer | Anoka, MN

"Not only do I 'like' this but I'm grateful that we started our concierge care two years ago.
It is yet another degree of peace-of-mind ...'
-Susan. | Connecticut

"I do not understand why you wouldn't do this. I can text my doctor and get a rapid response.
One time I had a rash. I took a picture of it with my iPhone, texted it to him and within a minute
he wrote me back and told me it should go away within two weeks."
-John | Pennsylvania

"I miss these kinds of doctors ..."
-Violette | Oklahoma

"Concierge Medicine is my savior. Love it!"
-Betty | San Diego, CA

"A fabulous alternative to the forced mechanisms of Obamacare!"
-Natalie | Atlanta, GA

"Not often does one have the opportunity to have this kind of doctor
that you feel is part of your life."
-Priscilla | Ohio

Legal Notice And Disclaimer

Intended Audience

This information is published for some, but not all the residents of the United States. This work is not intended for use outside of the United States of America.

Please Be Aware

While we make every effort to ensure that at the date of this book and its publication that the contact information below is up-to-date and accurate, we do recognize that the contact information, names, etc., are subject to change at any time. In addition to the resources, contacts, individuals and doctors mentioned in this book, we have provided you with a list of trusted physicians, resources, attorneys and businesses that you are welcome to reach out to at www.ConciergeMedicineToday.com or www.DirectPrimaryCare.com.

Table of Contents

INTRODUCTION
THE GREAT MISUNDERSTANDING.

THE JOY OF LEARNING.

CHAPTER 1
FOOLS RUSH IN. DO NOT QUIT YOUR DAY JOB, YET.

CHAPTER 2
GETTING STARTED.

THE ART of EDITING.

CHAPTER 3
PLANNING AND PREPARATION.

THE ART of EDITING (Con't).

CHAPTER 3 (Con't)
PLANNING AND PREPARATION.

CHAPTER 4
PUBLIC INTRODUCTION, PART 1.

THE JOB of MASTERING.

CHAPTER 5
PUBLIC INTRODUCTION, PART 2

Dramatic Decision-Making.

BENEFITS of HARVESTING.

CHAPTER 6
ARE WE THERE YET?

SATISFACTION IN GUIDING.

CHAPTER 7
RUNNING WITH THE GIANTS.

CHAPTER 8
YOUR JOURNEY BEGINS NOW.

- Six Traits Great Concierge Medicine and DPC Doctors Share.

SATISFACTION IN GUIDING (Con't).

CHAPTER 9
SUPPORTIVE INDUSTRY RESOURCES & CONTACTS

Introduction –
The Great Misunderstanding.

Why First Edition?

This First Edition is designed to be updated regularly. As businesses, rules, regulations and laws change, we plan to continue to update this body of work by printing and distributing later versions.

It is our hope that this Doctors Guidebook will educate you and your team about the various complexities, considerations and expectations you should have when entering this marketplace. This long awaited guidebook has already sold countless copies even prior to its printing. We have worked diligently over many years to make this book effective and educational. We trust you and your team will find it helpful. If so, please leave us a review on Amazon. We would greatly appreciate it!

Enjoy!

How To Use This Guidebook.

This guidebook is designed to answer questions regarding the various concerns, questions and processes surrounding the business of operating and/or starting a Concierge Medicine, retainer or DPC medical practice. It is designed specifically with the doctor and their staff in mind. It should furnish relevant, practical and helpful information to help you make many of the difficult decisions ahead of you.

Although the process and undertaking may appear intimidating due to its costs, complexity and sheer size and the number of topics covered, you will find it quite easy to use. The guidebook is subdivided into four main sections: Learning; Editing; Mastering, Harvesting and eventually, Guiding. Each chapter within each section targets a specific subject. Because of the diversity found in the various business models and operations seen in so many Concierge Medicine practices, we have included "Running With The Giants" an entire chapter highlighting the various success stories, how-to's and advice currently practicing concierge and DPC doctors have provided for others considering walking down the same path.

It is nearly impossible to find one size fits all process, let alone a guidebook that will explain everything to you. In all of our interviews, conversations and years of covering this industry and talking with countless physicians, consultants, staff administrators and franchise consultants, they will all advise any doctor or business person moving into this marketplace to surround yourself with a team. That team is further explained in later chapters in detail as well as the costs associated with transitioning a primary care or family medical practice into a Concierge Medicine, retainer-based practice or DPC medical clinic. Not all chapters of this guide will be applicable to any one business or doctor.

Physician Resources and Recommended Rules of Engagement.

Over the years, we have seen that there is a great resource shortage for physicians, business leaders and others desiring to learn more about this growing industry. The management team, industry contributors and writers at *Concierge Medicine Today* have worked to change all of that. Today, we are happy to provide the medical community with a wealth of resources, checklists, white papers, books, contacts, coaches, mentors and physician contacts to help you get your journey started. You can find many of these resources at our web site and online bookstore located at www.ConciergeMedicineToday.com.

Near the conclusion of this book, we have provided you with a list of physicians, resources, attorneys and businesses to which you may wish to reach out. Prior to contacting these resources, we advise the following:

1. Initially, please do not ask for more than 15 minutes of their time. You will probably end up with 30, but never ask for more than 15.
2. When making your request, we encourage you to ask your initial introductory request in terms of: 'I'd like to ask you about YOUR practice.' Not, 'I would like to ask you about MY practice.'
3. Please be as accommodating as possible. These individuals, businesses and others are 'on-the-clock' and have busy schedules. Please be courteous and grateful for their time.
4. Never ask one of the Physician Mentors or contributors to help you make your own business decisions. Consultants can help you make decisions. This is why Consultants get paid. The Physician Mentors mentioned in this guidebook will provide you with feedback, not make decisions for you.
5. Remember to listen more than you talk.
6. Ask questions!

"I'm always ready. I make house calls. I'll go to private offices –
whatever they need. I can do essentially anything that can be done
in most typical doctors' offices,"

~Dr. Robert Nelson, MyDoc~Personal Physician Services, Cumming, GA

"For I know the plans I have for you," declares the LORD, "plans to prosper you and not to harm
you, plans to give you hope and a future."

~Jeremiah 29:11 NIV

Addressing Myths and Common Obstacles.

"It is expensive."

That is the first thing I thought of years ago when I first learned about Concierge Medicine. When you dig a little deeper, the world and people around us share a very different story.

For busy parents, such as Charena and Lynn Swann, the convenience of a Concierge Doctor who treats their two adolescent sons at their home is too good to pass up. "We do not have to worry about going to a doctor's office where people are coughing and sick kids are playing with the same toys." said Charena Swann, 48, who lives in Sewickley, PA.

Today, this commonly misunderstood form of personalized-physician care is quickly reaching out to a massive audience of cost-conscious consumers across America. They understand that six minutes is not enough time to spend with their doctor. For a flat, out-of-pocket fee of $30 per month, Patients in one Michigan doctor's office have access to their doctor, diagnoses, disease management care, preventive care and many procedures right there at the doctors practice.

"I do not understand why you wouldn't do this," said John Kuntz, 52, an entrepreneur who lives in Collier, PA. "I can text my doctor and get a rapid response. One time I had a rash. I took a picture of it with my iPhone, texted it to him and within a minute he wrote me back and told me it should go away within two weeks."

Stories like the Swann Family and John's are typical concierge medical practice descriptions. If you think about it, Concierge Medicine is nothing new. It has been practiced by physicians for centuries. Today, this form of healthcare has been labeled concierge care. How expensive do you think the physician working in Andy Griffith's town of Mayberry was? Was he concerned about Medicare reimbursement for Aunt Bee? Did he ask Opie to schedule an office visit?

Today, false rhetoric surrounds the ethics and ideology of practicing Concierge Medicine physicians. Those who are not fans of the practice say it is a waste of money for the Patient. American culture is obsessed with the stories of high cost doctors who abandon their Patients in search of great riches. That almost sounds like something from an adventure story and is certainly a fabricated narrative.

I recently watched one local news station in the south interview a man who was clearly upset that his doctor of 18 months was changing his business model to accept monthly and annual memberships for healthcare.

"It is like paying for the privilege of seeing your doctor," said one former Patient to a television news reporter at WAFF in Huntsville, Alabama. "That just goes against everything I believe. I do not shop at Costco; I do not belong to Sam's Club. I do not believe in paying for the privilege of doing business with someone."

More often than not, these stories stop good doctors from even starting. Here are a few of the more common ones you might encounter:

- **MYTH: It is Only For The Rich.** For anyone earning between $20,000 and $80,000 dollars per year, Concierge Medicine is an affordable option. It is also a little known fact that most Concierge Doctors' office memberships (approx. 62% and growing) cost less than $135 per month. That is less than what most people pay for their cell phone or high-definition television service. Combine that cost with a high-deductible health plan policy or catastrophic wrap-around healthcare insurance plan and, more often than not, you will save money compared to years past.

- **MYTH: These Doctors Really Only Care About The Money.** If you have the heart to serve your Patients, this is an easy objection to overcome. If you truly believe it is more important to not have to look at a medical chart to know your Patient's name before turning the doorknob and entering the exam room, you will find a way to make it an affordable option. Conversely, if we really want that new car or that new addition added onto the house, you will find a way to afford it. As we will explain in the coming chapters, Concierge Medicine is one of the only medical models today in which doctors can forecast what their annual earnings will be. Would working in a medical practice like that be a better alternative than the late hours you are putting in now?

- **MYTH: My Patients Do not Make Enough To Afford It.** Patient income generally does not predict a concierge medical practice's rise or fall. Bedside manner (i.e. how much Patients actually like you and your staff), demographics, services offered, staff interactions, billing and promotion -- all of those factors contribute to the success or failure of a practice.

If it is because you dislike the current hamster-wheel healthcare system or Patient-doctor treadmill you are on and want to somehow strike back, there are more effective and cheaper ways to do it.

"Be clear why you want to do this," said Dr. Mitchell Karton, a Seattle, WA internist. "We never felt we were reacting adversarial against insurers. In fact, we remained on as many fee-for-services, PPO and POS panels as we could." [Dr. Karton and Dr. Garrison Bliss who together partnered to create Seattle Medical Associates years ago – a Patient-supported retainer-style practice]

When Patients Of Concierge Medical Care Were Asked Why They Choose Concierge Medical Care, They Said...

- 34% said price was the main reason they chose concierge medical care.
- 29% said insurance compatibility was the main reason they chose concierge medical care.
- 17% said Medicare acceptance/participation was the main reason they chose concierge medical care.
- 6% said more time with my doctor was the main reason they chose concierge medical care.
- 6% said less office staff to deal with was the main reason they chose concierge medical care.
- 2% said limited/no waiting was the main reason they chose concierge medical care.
- 6% indicated a variety of other reasons not included in the list above.

The takeaway here is that a lot of concierge practices focus on limited or no waiting at their office and not on the real issues driving Patients to these clinics, that being: insurance compatibility and price. While more time with the doctor and same day appointments are nice features of the practice, these were the least important aspects as to why Patients choose concierge medical care.

My Patients Hate The Idea of 'Concierge' Medicine.

I have spoken to dozens of doctors that cannot forget 'that one guy' or 'this one lady' who projected so much hate and negativity towards them when they asked the question that it made a lasting mental impression on them to this day. But, you do not know until you ask. You might find when you ask your Patients what they think of a monthly fee for enhanced access to their doctor is that some of your Patients were going to leave your practice in the next year because you are not able to spend enough time with them In fact, they have been wanting you to do something like this for months.

One concierge physician in North Carolina, Dr. John Kihm said "Patients who cannot see the value in your practice can and will vote with their feet. There is nothing unethical about letting Patients decide who they need."

In the upcoming Planning and Preparation Chapter, we will talk more about how to learn and discover what your Patients want from you and your practice before taking the leap into changing anything about your practice.

I Cannot Provide Around-The-Clock Care. When Will There
Be Time For A Vacation?

"I made the switch many years ago into Concierge Medicine, or at least a form of it, and couldn't be happier. I can provide better care and build a strong relationship with my Patients. It definitely can be challenging since I make myself available 24/7. However, if you can develop a good support structure of other like-minded MDs/DOs you can maintain a successful business with less stress than a traditional practice." ~*Las Vegas Urgent Care Clinic, January 2014*

According to surveys conducted by The Concierge Medicine Research Collective from 2009 to 2013, the question was asked of Concierge Doctors 'How often do your Patients call you after hours?' (i.e. 5pm-8am, Mon-Sun). The findings were surprising to a lot of people. Physicians received over 93% of their inquiries and calls from current Patients during normal business hours (9am-5pm). The vast majority of Patients knew their doctor and respected their physician's private and family life. Only in the event of severe emergencies were afterhours calls requested of the physician.

In the event you would like to take a vacation, it has never been easier to call a physician colleague, pay them a fair rate for their on-call time for your time away and tell them ... "I'm going on vacation for a week. I am going to give my Patients your number in the event they need a doctor's care. You will really enjoy them. They are very respectful and appreciate what we do as doctors by providing them with 24/7 service."

Dr. Thomas LaGrelius of SkyPark Medicine in Torrance, California says "You will never regret being a doctor IF you work ONLY for Patients. But if you do not work only for Patients, you will regret your decision in the end."

Is This Legal? What Are The Ethics?

The reality is that most doctors who practice traditional medicine in our current third-party payer system have a glaringly obvious conflict of interest. According to Dr. Steven Knope, 'They sign contracts with HMOs and insurance companies in exchange for Patient referrals from these companies. In many of these contracts, doctors agree to limit or ration care to Patients to maximize profits for these companies, their Wall Street shareholders and their CEOs. Some contracts even prevent the doctor from sharing this information with their Patients. By any reasonable assessment, this third-party payer system is intrinsically unethical. Concierge Medicine, by contrast, has no third-party conflicts. Patients pay their doctor directly for his services in the concierge model, just as they did in the days of Marcus Welby. In the concierge model, the doctor is the advocate for one party and one party only: the Patient. He/she has no allegiance to or conflicts with third parties.'

In most (approx.. 80%) concierge medical offices today, if you choose to accept insurance for some health plans and thus, file those claims with said insurer, your practice should be providing a technically non-covered service. If you pursue a career path in Concierge Medicine, you may hear some of your colleagues argue that by charging a fee, you limit access to Patients, thus, your way of doing business is not ethical.

For Dr. David Bisbee, the son of a seventh-generation Vermont dairy farmer, the motivation for switching to a concierge practice in late 2013 was only partly financial. The 59-year-old family practitioner says he was driven more by a desire to regain his "autonomy" as a physician and get back to the basics of why he got into medicine 27 years ago.

"I do house calls, I deliver babies, I go to the hospital and the nursing home," explains Bisbee, who is also the Medical Director of a long-term nursing facility in Morrisville. (He waives his annual fee for most of his elderly Patients and allows others to pay in installments.) "This is what I call a modern medical practice with a lot of old-fashioned notions."

Dr. Robert Nelson of MyDocPPS located in Cumming, GA notes "One cannot legislate or mandate professional ethics; a physician either possesses it or not. Physicians (providers) will NOT be more likely to put Patient welfare first in a third – party payer, heavily regulated system as compared to a system where the Patient also acts as the consumer, not just a passive recipient of care. In fact, the opposite is true. Our present system encourages providers to only do the minimum to satisfy audit requirements of payers. A consumer-driven system where the provider works FOR the Patient, not as a bill collector for the insurance company, would be MORE responsive to Patient needs and wishes; working with the Patient to establish an agreed upon level of care based on an informed Patient who is exercising choices allowed because they are both the consumer AND the Patient."

Donald O. Clifton said in the book *Now, Discover Your Strengths*' "There is one sure way to identify your greatest potential for strength: Step back and watch yourself for a while. Try an activity and see how quickly you pick it up, how quickly you skip steps in the learning and add twists and kinks you haven't been taught yet. See whether you become absorbed in the activity to such an extent that you lose track of time. If none of these has happened after a couple of months, try another activity and watch and then another. Over time your dominant talents will reveal themselves, and you can start to refine them into a powerful strength."

"Today the greatest single source of wealth is between your ears."
~Brian Tracy

"Cast all your anxiety on him because He cares for you."
~1 Peter 5:7 NIV

*"If you do not change the direction you are going,
then you are likely to end up where you are heading..."*
~John C. Maxwell

Transitioning My Practice To A Concierge Medicine Model Is Too
Expensive and Overwhelming!

"I love being an old school concierge doc and look forward to helping move this to the forefront of medicine to ultimately improve the health of all Americans!." ~Dr. Ronald Primas, New York

You are right. It is expensive. There are some individuals and businesses in the marketplace who at present, overcharging and underserving the physician and Patient communities. However, the marketplace is shifting and more, mentors, advisors, businesses and doctors now have more affordable choices to help them move into this space without breaking the bank.

We have been covering this industry for nearly a decade now. We have kept our eyes on many of the Concierge Doctors that have been operating since 1996. We have seen many succeed beyond their wildest dreams. At the same time, we have seen many Concierge Doctors' flounder. They have told us that operating and starting a concierge practice was not easy but it is rewarding. They are so glad they did it. Conversely, it is not an easy road to follow but, if done properly, it can be the most rewarding venture you will ever enter into.

The cost of franchise and consulting fees can move from five-figures and easily into six figures. According to *Concierge Medicine Today*, they have found the average cost is between $150,000 – $250,000 over a period of two to five years. In some rare cases, even longer. Some consultants have quoted figures less than $60,000. However, depending on your practice, it is the: demographics; your bedside manner; Patient surveys (very important); complexity of internal operations; a financial feasibility analysis; and many other variables that help determine whether a Concierge Medicine or DPC (DPC) practice may or may not be the right option for you.

"Perhaps most important from a doctors perspective," says industry DPC Consultant Mike Permenter, "is that a consulting company should typically furnish all of the capital required to start or modify your medical practice and assumes all risk for success of failure. Thus, the high fees. My fees are much different than the industry standard."

As with most of the companies operating in the Concierge Medicine marketplace, a doctor (i.e. franchisee) will pay an ongoing periodic royalty fee. CMT has found this to be as low as 15% of each Patient's individual membership fee but, in most cases, is between 29% to 33% for a period of approximately 3 to 5 years. In some rare cases, up to 25% of your per Patient fee for eight years has been reported to CMT by doctors considering a transition to Concierge Medicine or DPC. These fees usually include continued support and training in: advertising; marketing; sales; operational guidance; technology; legal; regulatory; financial and human resources consulting; along with other critical services.

You Need To Reach Out For Help.

"Business is tough," says Dr. Chris Ewin of 121MD in Fort Worth, TX. "If you are doing something just for the money, you are never going to enjoy it. You will be the hardest boss you have ever had. So, find something you love and pursue it. Follow this advice and you will set yourself up for an enjoyable future in medicine."

If you think you can do this alone, think again. You need staff that supports you (and believes in what your new practice model stands for), a spouse that thinks you should do this and advice from a great accountant, a trusted attorney, a consultant and a few savvy business people to help guide you along the way.

Never ask a Physician Mentor or colleague of yours in this industry to help you make your own business decisions when starting your concierge or DPC medical practice. Consultants can help you make decisions. This is why Consultants get paid. The Physician Mentors mentioned in this guidebook may provide you with feedback, but they should not make decisions for you.

In the coming chapters, it is our hope that you will begin to prioritize your passions. Find an enthusiasm buried down deep for practicing medicine apart from paperwork and frustrating insurance hassles. It is not easy. We will not promise you overnight success. Someone once said 'overnight successes take 10 years.' It probably won't take you that long. It is likely that more physicians, especially physicians in smaller practices, will begin transitioning to Concierge Medicine around you. Even more direct-pay/retail medical clinics may spring up in the coming years in your local area. They probably already have and you are just not aware of it. Physicians who favor independent practice will likely view these alternative reimbursement models as a way to retain their independence, spend more time with Patients, and combat declining reimbursement, enabling them to continue to practice medicine as they have desired.

Lastly, please note, we are not rendering legal, accounting or other professional advice in this book. It is up to the individual or business owner to seek out the advice of competent professionals to assist them in decision making.

Dr. Thomas LaGrelius of SkyPark Medicine in Torrance, California says
"You will never regret being a doctor IF you work only for Patients.
But if you do not work only for Patients, you will regret your decision in the end."

Chapter 1 –
The Art of Learning.

Fools Rush In. Do not Quit Your Day Job, Yet.

A Vision Is Born. You Are Here.

"When doctors talk about Concierge Medicine being "the oldest, new form of medicine," they are not speaking figuratively—they are trying to reframe the identity of their practice in an over-worked industry." ~Catherine Sykes, Publisher, Author, Speaker, The DPC Journal

We all have great visions and big dreams for our lives. At one time or another, we have all probably had an idea for a million dollar invention that someone else eventually developed and brought to market. Now, years later, they live on the interest from earnings somewhere in a mansion or on a yacht

You have probably had the same experience or met someone who invented something so simple and so obvious that you thought 'I could have done that in my sleep.' You could be that millionaire now too. But what happened? Why did you talk yourself out of that one good idea that could have altered the trajectory of your life? You probably thought to yourself, 'How come he thought of that and I didn't?!' The answer is, you may have thought of that idea but because you are too smart, you talked yourself out of pursuing the idea through to its entirety. The idea of a doctor who sees us without delay, returns phone calls promptly, sends us emails, video chats or receives texts is completely foreign. The same can be said about the need for Concierge Medicine, DPC healthcare and listing your fee(s) like popular fast-food chains do in your own local medical community. However, doctors doing exactly this work in offices across the country and are providing their Patients with affordable access and services.

Think about where you are in the business of medicine today. Are you happy? How did you get here? Why are you really reading this book? You have stumbled upon or learned about this book because you are most likely in a learning phase in your business or life. You need to know 'what is next?' This is not simply an intellectual exercise; this is an emotional and business decision that is going to change your life and that of your Patients and family.

The truth is Concierge Medicine is now a lifeline for a growing number of doctors frustrated with America's healthcare system. Jon Acuff writes in his book *Start: Punch Fear in the Face, Escape Average and Do Work that Matters*, as people in our careers, we must go through very distinct stages or phases in life to become masters of our business. He writes that 'Nothing cripples your business, budget or causes more frustration that spending money and not seeing results, right?' Overcoming fear and the success that follows is learned, edited and shortly thereafter, mastered.

To know what to expect before you start, you must understand that choosing a career in Concierge Medicine is not for the faint-hearted. It requires vision and hopefully, that is where you are today. Doctors tell us every day at *Concierge Medicine Today* that this chosen career path is one of the most challenging they have ever faced, especially the first 18-months. The reward however, is completely worth it.

Finding Career Fulfillment

"This new practice has been truly liberating. I am working harder than ever getting it off the ground but my time with Patients is wonderful. And I get to be creative again in how I develop the practice, something that was lost from my previous office." ~Dr. Alicia Cunningham, Vermont

You are among friends here. The community of physicians and healthcare professionals you are about to learn about are spread out across the U.S. What they will tell you is that they are actually happy with their career in Concierge Medicine, DPC and cash-only medicine in some form. Imagine that, feeling happy about your practice at the end of the day. When your spouse looks at you after a hard day at the practice and notices that the weight of your business is lifted, that is worth every penny. Pursuing a path in Concierge Medicine is less about what the media tells you and more about relief in the eyes of your Patients and your staff when they tell you, 'Only 6 appointments today.'

Career satisfaction among physicians in this field remains high. According to *The Concierge Medicine Research Collective* (www.AskTheCollective.org), the research and data collection arm of the industry's trade journal and news outlet, *Concierge Medicine Today*, only 18% of physicians stated they would not make the same decision again. In previous years, it was as high as 25% but even so, the number overall is low and satisfaction with the business model is high when compared to traditional, insurance-based or managed care business models. In 2012, approximately 55% of Concierge Doctors across the U.S. stated they are *very satisfied* with their decision to enter Concierge Medicine and would make the same decision. 27% of Concierge Doctors are somewhat satisfied with their decision to enter Concierge Medicine but would make the same decision.

Concierge Medicine and DPC medical practice are career paths physicians can trust. Over time, they have proven to be sustainable and rewarding business models for both physicians and his or her Patients. But to do this, and to do it right, is about being focused, strategic and following a gradual process that begins with learning ... baby steps, if you will.

We can confidently tell you from the countless interviews, stories and advice we have given to doctors over the years is that you are about to embark on a journey that is going to change the trajectory of your life, your career and help people more than you could ever imagine.

"The best way to find out whether you are on the right path? Stop looking at the path."
~Marcus Buckingham

"I can do all things through Christ who strengthens me."
~Philippians 4:13 NKJV

What Is Concierge Medicine?

Concierge Medicine is a form of membership in which doctors provide medical care to Patients generally providing 24/7 access, a cell phone number to connect directly with their physician, same-day appointments, visits that last as long as it takes to address their needs and varying other amenities. In exchange for this enhanced access and personal attention, the Concierge Doctor receives a fee (most fees average between $135-$150/mo., Source: ConciergeMedicineToday.com, 2014) which enables them to increase the amount of time they spend with Patients.

"We are a family of mom, dad, and 10 year old daughter," says a mother in Marietta, GA. "Dad's retirement from his job means leaving his insurance plan. We are healthy and looking for affordable DPC Medical Care or Concierge Care."

A Concierge Doctor becomes the source for all things medical. Essentially, you become a trusted friend, advocate and stand fully prepared to help your Patients navigate the complex healthcare system. In the event of emergencies, hospital care is closely monitored, and specialists are often personally briefed and debriefed by you on behalf of your Patients.

"Even if you (a Patient) have insurance, you still do not have access to care," says Dr. Chris Ewin or 121MD in Dallas/Fort Worth, TX. "You can have all the insurance you want. You still cannot get in to see the doctor."

This is why thousands of people are now actively searching for a Concierge Doctor or a DPC physician. They also discover that out-of-pocket costs to this type of doctor can actually save them thousands of dollars a year. At the same time, they can have their doctor's cell phone on speed dial.

What Is DPC?

DPC (DPC) clinics or DPC doctors, similar to Concierge Medicine, is another popular emerging business model. Patients pay one low monthly fee, sometimes as low as $49-$99/mo. directly to their DPC physician for all of their everyday health needs. Like a health club membership, this fee (avg. $50-$99/indiv.) provides Patients with unrestricted access to visits and care. Patients can use the services as much or as little as they want. Many DPC practices are open seven days per week and offer same-day or next-day appointments. At many clinics, physicians are on call 24/7.

"This primary care business model [DPC] gives these types of providers the time to deliver more personalized care to their Patients and pursue a comprehensive medical home approach," said a spokesperson at Qliance Medical Management based in Seattle, Washington. "... The provider's incentives are fully aligned with the Patient's incentives."

With DPC, there are no insurance co-pays, deductibles or co-insurance fees. DPC doctors do not typically accept insurance payments, thus avoiding the overhead and complexity of maintaining relationships with insurers. This can save significant overhead expense as managing insurance relationships can consume as much as $0.40 of each medical dollar spent.

DPC practices typically have monthly membership fees under $100 and serve a population of households earning $70,000 or less, according to *The Concierge Medicine Research Collective*. Monthly Concierge Medicine membership fees usually are slightly higher, about $135 per month and can include more in-office services. Despite the cost advantage, the DPC model may be hampered by low awareness among health plans and primary care physicians, resistance from some insurers, and resistance from competing hospitals and specialists. Although, significant efforts are underway to accelerate the DPC movement, so this disadvantage may disappear as awareness grows.

In a report published by the California HealthCare Foundation, five large DPC clinics in the U.S. using a DPC healthcare service model serve over 500,000 lives. These charge either direct fees paid to the doctor, the physicians practice, or via self-insured employers and health plans.

Overall, Concierge Medicine and DPC style clinics are thriving in major metropolitan markets. Of great benefit to the consumers, prices are dropping dramatically due to increasing competition among physicians entering the marketplace, retail medicine pricing, price transparency demand from Patients and continued uncertainty about the implications of the Affordable Care Act.

The Difference Between Concierge Medicine and DPC

DPC (DPC) is a term often linked to its companion in health care, 'Concierge Medicine.' Although the two terms are similar and belong to the same family, Concierge Medicine is a term that fully embraces or 'includes' many different health care delivery models, DPC being one of them.

Similarities

DPC practices, similar in philosophy to their Concierge Medicine lineage – typically bypass insurance and go for a more 'direct' financial relationship with Patients.. They also provide comprehensive care and preventive services for an affordable fee. However, DPC is only one branch in the family tree of Concierge Medicine.

Similar to concierge health care practices, DPC removes many of the financial barriers to accessing care whenever it is needed. There are generally no co-pays, deductibles or co-insurance fees. DPC practices also do not typically accept insurance payments, thus avoiding the overhead and complexity of maintaining relationships with insurers, which can consume as much as $0.40 of each medical dollar spent (Sources: Dave Chase and California Health Foundation).

Under most Patient-physician contracts in DPC and concierge medical clinics, Patients (and workers at employer groups, small and mid-size businesses) pay no co-pay for services. In addition to the services that the doctor provides on-site and inside the practice, individuals and companies maintain lower cost insurance plans to accommodate major medical expenditures and more intensive procedures. In that sense, the model for healthcare is similar to that being pursued by many internal medicine, specialty physicians and family practitioners, who are today, reducing their Patient load by two-thirds, dropping insurance wrangling and adopting a DPC model paid with an (almost) all-inclusive, monthly, quarterly or annual subscription fee.

Differences

According to a spokesperson at Qliance Medical Management based in Seattle, Washington, DPC is a 'mass-market variant of Concierge Medicine, distinguished by its low prices.' Simply stated, the biggest difference between 'DPC' and retainer based practices is that DPC generally takes a low, flat rate fee whereas concierge models plans usually charge a slightly higher annual retainer fee and promise more time spent with a doctor. Also, services in concierge models tend to more service-focused and added-value oriented versus just providing access and more convenience to the practice.

"This primary care business model [DPC] gives these type of providers the time to deliver more personalized care to their Patients and pursue a comprehensive medical home approach," said Norm Wu, CEO of Qliance Medical Management based in Seattle, Washington. "One in which the provider's incentives are fully aligned with the Patient's incentives."

A History of Concierge Medicine. Bringing History Back To Life.

Doctors carrying a medical bag and coming into a Patient's home was standard into the late 1960s. Look at The Andy Griffith Show. Remember Marcus Welby, MD? That is what our grandparents know. Medicine became more and more government and insurance regulated and that started to end. It came in for a reason -- there did need to be some amount of administration. But now regulation and administrative tasks have frustrated doctors.

2013 and 2014 were some the most eventful years in the space of Concierge Medicine, private-pay and DPC as news and headlines continued to circulate across the wire. From *The New York Times* to *The Wall Street Journal* and everywhere in between, Concierge Medicine was becoming a familiar term that people are beginning to understand as an affordable healthcare option. *Concierge Medicine Today* and its sister-publication, *The DPC Journal* covered this industry and reached millions of new readers, Patients and others with headlines now being read regularly in over 130 countries and inside thousands of medical offices and homes across the U.S.

*"Hope deferred makes the heart sick,
but a longing fulfilled is a tree of life."*
-Proverbs 13:12 NIV

"People who produce good results feel good about themselves."
-Ken Blanchard

Why would I want to consider practicing in a Concierge Medicine, retainer or DPC practice?

"The road was much more difficult than I expected, but also much more satisfying. I spent much of my time learning what does not work, but in the end learned that most good ideas grow out of the remains of a hundred bad ones that didn't survive." ~ DPC Physician, Rob Lamberts, MD, Augusta, GA

Most doctors that subscribe to our publication already understand and know the value this type of business model offers to their practice, Patients, staff, family and lifestyle. However, for those that are wondering, one of the most appealing aspects of the various Concierge Medicine and DPC business models is that the retainer fee payment structure can greatly simplify the business of operating a primary care and/or family practice. These types of practices report significantly reduced operating overhead when compared with traditional, managed-care primary care and family practice environments. This is primarily due to the large number of these practices that do not need to maintain dedicated staff to organize, review, file, and manage payment from and claims to third-party payers.

Approximately 20% of these types of medical practices do not participate in contracts with private insurance carriers at all. The physician community calls this business model 'DPC (DPC).' They avoid the economic pressures of declining reimbursements provided by most managed care organizations. Also important to note, Concierge Medicine and retainer-based medical practices that do choose to continue participating in their insurance carrier contracts, continue to accept private insurance. The simplification of practice administration, appointment scheduling and billing processes has resulted in an improved work-life balance for these physicians. Currently, approximately 80% according to surveys from The Concierge Medicine Research Collective, act in a far more proactive manner and only participate in insurance contracts that are economically beneficial for the practice and the Patient.

Last, many primary care and family doctors practicing in Concierge Medicine settings report that these models afford the opportunity to spend more time with Patients. This has resulted in improved professional satisfaction. This anecdotal evidence is bolstered by reduced hospitalizations, greater prescription compliance and healthier physician evaluations.

Four Noteworthy Occurrences In 2013 That Are Worth Mentioning.

First, Patient interest hit an all-time high as more and more prospective and curious Patients started to enroll in Concierge Medicine and DPC (DPC) practices. CMT reports that January thru April of 2014 had the highest amount of Patient enrollments in these practices.

"We have certainly seen an increase in physician interest," says Catherine Sykes, publisher and Managing Director of *The DPC Journal (The DPC Journal)*. "Our opinion and that of our research arm, *The Concierge Medicine Research Collective*, is that there are approximately 12,000+ physicians participating in these models nationwide."

Also a noteworthy point related to Patient and consumer interest is the amount of books sold this year by Concierge Medicine Today's Bookstore. Three books in particular are selling faster than inventory can be kept in stock. *The Patient Guide To Concierge Medicine and DPC Practices* is now being distributed through doctors' offices to prospective Patients as an educational tool to help physicians and their staff educate, persuade and guide Patients into making a decision about DPC and Concierge Medicine practices for them and their family. In 2013, *Branding Concierge Medicine, Volume I.*, reached the top 2% of all Amazon and Kindle eBooks across the country.

"The distinctions between Concierge Medicine, private medicine, and DPC may be ultimately meaningless, since some doctors call themselves whatever they feel sounds better, and there are so many practice variations, many overlapping, that it often isn't clear which is which." ~Neil Chesanow, Medscape/WebMD, May 2014

Second, the power of the media in America has crowned their winning brand name and it is the term "Concierge Medicine." Like it, hate it or simply indifferent to it, the term appeared in headlines and stories over 106,450 times alone in 2013.

The use of the term, controversial and often misunderstood is a brand name and houschold term that the media adopted from among a wide variety of options such as: boutique medicine; retainer medicine; wealth-care; cash-only medicine, etc. Not to be confused with its familiar cousin, DPC (DPC), Concierge Medicine is a slightly different type of doctors office with different services offered than its often aligned, DPC term. Concierge Medicine is now widely understood to be a real healthcare alternative and growing option for the middle-class Patient and Mom-types. So, get used to the brand and term ... it is here to stay.

In a story in January 2014, one reporter writes ... despite the name "Concierge Medicine," local physicians think the model is accessible to those with lower incomes.

"Good understanding brings forth favor ..."
~Proverbs 13:15 NIV

Third, DPC clinics or DPC doctors, similar to their healthcare cousin, Concierge Medicine, emerged in a big way in 2013. The first-ever DPC Conferences were held in St. Louis, MO in October 2013 and June 2014 in Washington, D.C. More events and DPC meetings are slated to occur in 2015 and beyond.

The practice of DPC is growing, but the web of providers is so fragmented that even those in the field do not know how many physicians or practices work in this way, said Sharon George, MD, who owns a one-physician DPC practice in Irvine, Calif.

"It is definitely growing," she added. "You do not have to leave medicine if you are frustrated. You have your medical degree."

The DPC Coalition formed as Congress was debating the Affordable Care Act (ACA). At that time, the coalition estimated there were between 30 and 50 single and multi-physician practice locations in the U.S., with around 100,000 Patients.

But Erika Bliss, MD, told *MedPage Today* that it is likely there are more Concierge Doctors -- and Patients who use their services -- practicing today.

Bliss, a leader of the coalition and chief executive of the five-location concierge practice Qliance, based in Seattle, said she receives Google alerts monthly about a new concierge practice or converting practice, and estimated one DPC practice in nearly every state in 2013.

Fourth, the first, Medical Centers Concierge Alliance Conference targeting Hospital Physicians, Administrators and Medical Center Executives was held in Seattle, WA in August of 2013. The Dare Center of Seattle, WA invited concierge physicians, hospital administrators and medical center executives from across the country who participated in a roundtable discussion. At least 20 medical centers were represented at this meeting.

There was a breakout session for program managers in established practices and another for attendees exploring this type of practice model. Topics also included: alternative models; amenities/perks; preserving academic standards; legal hurdles; marketing tips; compensation issues; expectations/boundaries; recruiting; networking and other topics of interest.

Brief And Abridged History Of Concierge Medicine And The DPC Healthcare Marketplace.

1996: Dr. Howard Maron and Scott Hall, FACP established MD2 (pronounced MD squared) located in Seattle, Bellevue, WA and Oregon. They charged an annual retainer fee of $13,200 and $20,000 per family.

1999: Medical Professionalism Project-consisting of members of the internal medicine community, including representatives of ACP and the American Board of Internal Medicine, set out to draft a charter that could serve as a framework for understanding professionalism.

1999:   Institute of Medicine releases the now famous report of medical errors, Patient safety, and professional integrity that caused further probing in physician exam rooms.

2000:   Virginia Mason Medical Center in Seattle, WA began operating concierge medical services within its facilities and used some of the profits from the 5 physician practice to subsidize other programs and indigent care services.

2000:   MDVIP, founded by Dr. Robert Colton and Bernard Kaminetsky, in Boca Raton, FL. A brand of Concierge Medicine practice and management firm which has set-up more than 700 concierge medical practices with offices in almost every State across the U.S. Update: In April 2014, Procter & Gamble announced the sale of MDVIP to a private equity firm, Summit Partners.

2001:   American Medical Association writes concierge physician guidelines: PRINCIPLES OF MEDICAL ETHICS.

2002:   ACB Foundation , ABIM Foundation and the European Federation of Internal Medicine defines ethical principles and responsibilities contracts between Patient and physician, which is in a language that suggests both parties have equality, mutual interest and autonomy.

2002:   Medicare addresses Concierge Medicine and retainer fees.

2002:   Centers for Medicare and Medicaid, CMS, outlined its position on concierge care in a March 2002 memorandum. The memorandum states that physicians may enter into retainer agreements with their Patients as long as these agreements do not violate any Medicare requirements.

2002:   Pinnacle Care establishes Patient care with a one-time membership fee for access to VIP service.

2002:   The AMA counsel on medical services issued a report in June 2002 on Special Physician-Patient contracts. It concluded that retainer medicine was a very small phenomenon.

2003:   American Society of Concierge Physicians was founded by Dr. John Blanchard. The association later changed its name to SIMPD, Society for Innovative Practice Design.

2003:   AMA issued guidelines for boutique practices in June 2003.

2003:   Department of Health and Human Services rules the concierge medical practices are not illegal and the federal government the OIG, Office of the Inspector General, takes a decidedly hands off approach.

2003:   American College of Physicians writes doctors struggle to balance professionalism with the pressures of everyday practice.

"We recognized back in 2000 that health care was moving from personal to a more institutionalized form, and it was not what we wanted to do. We felt we needed to have time with our Patients, to have the excellence to have the time with Patients. Health care has been cutting reimbursement to doctors, which has forced doctors to see more Patients, so the time doctors have with their Patients has declined. The average time today with Patients for most doctors is only 10 minutes."

-Dr. John Blanchard of Premier Private Physicians,
Troy and Clarkston, Michigan.

2003: June 2003 the AMA Council on Ethical and Judicial Affairs outlines guidelines for "contracted medical services". The AMA House of Delegates approves these guidelines.

2004: GAO, General Accountability Office writes 146 concierge physicians in the U.S.

2004: Harvard University study finds that 55% of the respondents are dissatisfied with their health care, and 40% of that 55% agreed that the quality of care had worsened in the previous five years.

2005: The AOA, American Osteopathic Association adopts not to recommend and an official policy on concierge care.

2006: MDVIP, a concierge physician practice management firm, reports that 130 physicians within their network treat up to 40,000 Patients worldwide.

2007: *Concierge Medicine Today*, a concierge medical news agency opens its doors to be an advocate for news pertaining to the Concierge Medicine, retainer-based, boutique, private medicine and direct care industry.

2007: The term "direct practice" was first used in legislation in Washington in 2007 that clarified these practices were not insurance companies under state law-but they do provide basic, preventive medical care.

2008: Boasting an estimated 35 concierge physician practices, Orange County, CA appeared to be a leading hub of Concierge Medicine.

2008: Concierge Physician of Orange County (CPOC)– a non-profit group of existing concierge physicians was founded.

2009: *Concierge Medicine Today*, announces the formation of The Concierge Medicine Research Collective.

2009: *Concierge Medicine Today*, reveals that concierge medical practices across the U.S. are thriving in a recession.

2009: Procter & Gamble Acquired MDVIP in 2009 - No less a respected corporation than Procter & Gamble (NYSE: PG) has staked out a major presence in Concierge Medicine. In 2007, P&G acquired a 48% stake in MDVIP, a Concierge Medicine company that was formed in 2000. Then, in December 2009, Procter & Gamble acquired 100% ownership in MDVIP for an undisclosed sum. This acquisition was reported by Dark Daily. (See "Boutique Medicine Venture Generates Marketing Intelligence for Procter & Gamble," April 5, 2010.)

2010: SIMPD reorganizes, expands its vision, and rebrands itself the American Academy of Private Physicians (AAPP).

2010:   *Concierge Medicine Today*, reveals the affordability of concierge medical and private medicine practices across the U.S. stating that over 62% of the programs offered to Patients cost less than $135/mo.

2010:   American Academy of Private Physicians (AAPP) forms first local chapter in Orange County, California called AAPP,OC (formerly CPOC)

2010:   According to a 2010 American Academy of Family Physicians survey, three percent of respondents practice in a cash-only, direct care, concierge, boutique, or retainer medical practice.

2012:   December 2012 - Study Proves Dramatic Reduction in Hospitalizations & $300 Million Savings for MDVIP's Personalized Healthcare Model

2013:   Three Year Analysis of Concierge and Direct Care Medicine Shows Encouraging Signs For Boosting Primary Care In U.S. Economy. Data collected from Concierge Medicine and DPC doctors show encouraging signs across the U.S. from December of 2009 to December of 2012.

2013:   New Data on Concierge Medicine Physician and DPC (DPC) Clinician Salaries and Released by Concierge Medicine Today. Data also looks at career satisfaction among Concierge/DPC physicians.

2013:   On August 2, 2013, the Dare Center, Seattle, WA, invited concierge physicians, hospital administrators and medical center executives from across the country to participate in a roundtable discussion. This inaugural event took place at the Washington Athletic Club in Seattle.

2013:   Family Physicians, Patients Embrace DPC ... AAFP Recognizes Benefits, Creates DPC Policy

2013:   *The DPC Trade Journal* Launched. *The DPC Journal* works directly and indirectly with physicians, businesses and leaders, journalists and the media in the healthcare marketplace to help promote the distribution of news and information, policy initiatives and to reach out to physicians throughout the United States. www.DirectPrimaryCare.com.

2013:   First National Gathering Focused On DPC (DPC) Held In St. Louis: October 11-12, 2013.

"This is the first national gathering of businesses and individuals interested in DPC," says Dr. Erika Bliss, a Family Physician at Qliance Medical Group of WA and President/CEO of Qliance Medical Management Inc. "DPC is quickly becoming an important contributor to the transformation of our nation's healthcare system. This conference will bring together key stakeholders to learn more about DPC and discuss its place in the future of medical care delivery."

"The DPC National Summit will bring together physicians, business leaders, policymakers and others from across the country," added Bliss. "DPC providers and supporters share the common goal of contributing meaningfully to the improvement of healthcare for all, and by building connections among like-minded people, we hope to accelerate progress toward that goal."

Overall, Concierge Medicine and DPC are thriving in major metropolitan markets. Four states that have a huge lead in the amount of active concierge or private-pay physician's in practice as well as consumers seeking their care are: Florida, California, Pennsylvania and Virginia. Each of these States have a significant number of people, most are over the age of 50, seeking out Concierge Doctors and cash-only options. Fortunately, a sizeable number of Concierge Doctors are available to serve them, which is not the case in the more rural parts of the country. In these states is where we are seeing franchise Concierge Medicine fees increase and independent Concierge Doctor fees decrease due to increasing competition and Patient demand for more price transparency.

Of great benefit to consumers, prices are dropping significantly due to increasing competition among physicians entering the marketplace, retail medicine pricing, price transparency demand from Patients and uncertainty about the implications of the Affordable Care Act. The Affordable Care Act has also created quite a bit of uncertainty among both Patients and doctors. The shoe has most certainly dropped and now more doctors than ever are considering a career in Concierge Medicine, DPC and retail healthcare.

2014: New Association Formed, American College of Private Physicians (ACPP): Group to Focus on Credentialing Doctors, Advocacy to Employers, Unions, Government and the like to benefit industry nationwide.

2014: P&G sells concierge medicine unit: P&G CEO — 'Since returning as CEO last year, A.G. Lafley has said P&G will exit ventures that won't help it grow.'

2014: MDVIP to be Acquired by Summit Partners — 'MDVIP will continue to be run as a stand-alone company ...' [May 2, 2014]

2014: IRS asked to clarify HSA rules in letter: On June 17, 2014, Members of Congress wrote Commissioner of Internal Revenue John Koskinen asking for clarification on how the Internal Revenue Service (IRS) treats DPC Medical Homes with regard to Health Savings Accounts (HSAs). Senator Maria Cantwell (D-WA), who authored ACA Sec. 1301 (a) (3), allowing DPC practices to participate in health exchanges with Qualified Health Plans, took the lead on the letter and was joined by Senate Budget Committee Chairman Patty Murray (D-WA) and Rep. Jim McDermott, MD (D-WA), ranking member of the Ways and Means Subcommittee on Health. The three WA state lawmakers point out that The ACA rules on the Establishment of Exchanges and Qualified Health Plans Part I (CMS-9989-F) promulgated by HHS, clearly state that DPC is not health insurance, and that the law has its roots in a provision in WA state law (48.150RCW) defining DPC as a health benefit outside insurance. IRS Continues to give guidance that DPC plans are considered health plans under Sec. 223 (c) of the Internal Revenue Code (IRC), which prohibits HSA account holders with high deductible health plans from having a second "health plan." DPC members have met with officials in the Department of the Treasury and continue to work with the administration and Congress to change the IRS definition so that DPC fees are qualified medical expenses under Sec. 213 (d) of the IRC and can be offered as a benefit complimenting Health Savings Accounts (HSAs) paired with high deductible health plans.

2014:   Second National Gathering Focused On DPC (DPC) Held In Wash., DC., June 2014.

2014: DPC United, a new DPC Physician Association, launched by Dr. Samir Qamar of MedLion announces that it will provide resources for DPC physicians and consumers.

2014: Michigan DPC Bill Introduced as Louisiana Passes Law: On September 9, 2014, Michigan State Senator Patrick Colbeck (R-Canton) introduced S.B. 1033, a bill to amend the MI state insurance code to clarify that a DPC agreement is not subject to state insurance regulation. DPCC has provided resourced to Sen. Colbeck, and we are watching developments in state legislatures around the country as they prepare for the coming sessions.   This summer, Gov. Bobby Jindal (R-LA) signed similar legislation; Senate Bill No. 516, making Louisiana the latest state to create law to define DPC practices correctly outside the scope of insurance regulation.   Stay tuned for further updates as the legislative sessions kick off in this coming January.

2014:   DPCC member Iora health recently announced an exciting new partnership with Humana to treat Medicare Advantage patients in Washington and Arizona. According to the Iora release, "The partnership launches Iora's unique health care model in Arizona and Washington where Iora Health will open four new primary care practices – two in Phoenix and two in Seattle – under the Iora Primary Care brand. The primary care practices are designed exclusively for Humana's Medicare Advantage members and will provide members access to affordable, quality care."

2014: New Study Conducted by Optum and MDVIP Finds Personalized Preventive Care Significantly Reduces Healthcare Expenditures Among Medicare Advantage Beneficiaries

2014:   September 2014, American Academy of Private Physicians (AAPP) Course Corrects Physician Association, citing that the industry's association is focusing on five key areas. Those include: legal compliance for doctors, innovative learning tracks at national meetings, physician networking, legislative and lobbying initiatives and staying up to date on new and emerging technologies..

Your ability to withstand the pressure and overcome the obstacles of uncertainty
and potential failure and see the other side before others do is what makes a successful concierge
[direct-pay] physician ...

"There are no insurance codes for 'cure,'" says
Dr. Garrison Bliss of Qliance, based in Seattle, WA.

2014: In October 2014, at the AAFP Assembly, a DPC Track is added to the agenda in Washington, D.C. It was called the "Health is Primary" initiative, a key business model for success touted by the AAFP (American Academy of Family Physicians).

2014: Washington State OIC issued DPC Outlook in Washington State. The OIC report insinuated that DPC is losing ground in terms of patients and that our monthly fees have been climbing (presumably as we head toward concierge medicine pricing).

2014: In reply, The DPC Journal assimilated a DPC leadership response to the Washington State OIC Report publishing for legislators, payers, physicians and the like: 'DPC Leadership Response To Washington State OIC Report: 'Outlook for DPC is bright throughout U.S.'

2014: *The DPC Journal* releases its industry-wide definition of DPC, the *5-Minute Guide: What Makes DPC Different From Concierge Medicine.* Also releases 2-Year analysis of DPC marketplace data.

2015: Michigan State Sen. Pat Colbeck, R-Canton, believes the path to providing Michigan citizens with access to higher quality, lower cost health care has been cleared following Gov. Rick Snyder's signature into law of Colbeck's SB 1033 (Public Act 522 of 2014). The new law in Michigan assures physicians who adopt a direct primary care service business model that the administrative burden associated with insurance regulations will not interfere with their treatment of patients. Physicians who offer direct primary care services provide specified services for a monthly subscription fee that usually vary between $50 and $125 per month. States with DPC Laws: Source: DPCare.org; Current as of January 22, 2015: Washington – 48-150 RCW; Utah – UT 31A-4-106.5; Oregon – ORS 735.500; West Virginia- WV-16-2J-1; Arizona – S.B. 1404; Louisiana – S.B. 516; Michigan – S.B. 1033

2014: *Specialdocs,* a pioneer and leading Concierge Medicine consulting firm says 'Cardiology, Endocrinology, Pulmonology, Pediatrics and OB GYN Practices Can Benefit from Conversion to Concierge Model.'

2015: The United Hospital Fund Releases A Report, *Convenient Care: Retail Clinics and Urgent Care Centers In New York State.*

This report is relevant to Concierge Care and the DPC healthcare space because: Although based on a small sample from a single group practice in Minnesota, the study found that patients who visited retail clinics had lower total costs than matched patients who visited the acute care clinic (Rohrer, Angstman, and Bartel 2009). A more recent study of adult primary care patients, also in Minnesota, found that the odds of return visits for treatment of sinusitis were the same whether patients received care at a retail clinic or in a regular office visit (Rohrer, Angstman, and Garrison 2012).

Perhaps more telling, a larger study of spending patterns of CVS Caremark employees found a significantly lower total cost of care in the year following a first visit to a retail clinic compared to costs incurred by propensity score-matched individuals who received care in other settings. In total, retail clinic users spent $262 less than their counterparts, with savings stemming primarily from lower medical expenses at physicians' offices ($77 savings) and reduced spending for hospital inpatient care ($121 savings). Retail clinic users also had 12 percent fewer emergency department visits than their counterparts (Sussman et al. 2013). The UHF saw nothing analogous on the impact of urgent care centers on total costs, but one study found that initial use of an urgent care center significantly reduced emergency department visits without increasing patient hospitalizations (Merritt, Naamon, and Morris 2000). Those results should be cautiously interpreted, however, given the study's design limitations.

Conversely, in September 2014, the MDVIP model also was shown to have saved some $3.7 million in reduced medical utilization for the 2,300 MDVIP Medicare Advantage patients over two years. Savings were $86.68 per patient per month in year one, and $47.03 per patient per month in year two, compared with patients who did not join an MDVIP practice. The two-year study explored preventive healthcare's ability to improve outcomes by creating a closer, personalized physician-patient relationship and focusing on disease prevention for Medicare Advantage.

2015: PinnacleCare, a leading health advisory firm, studied the impact of an expert second opinion on medical outcomes.

Researchers collected data on 1,000 cases on a three-year period and found that almost 77 percent of medical interventions led to changes in diagnosis, treatment, and/or treating physician. PinnacleCare gathered data on patient outcomes from their interventions over a three-year period. In a sampling of 1,000 cases with known outcomes from 2012-2014, 41% resulted in transfer of care to a COE or expert provider with 34% resulting in a change in diagnosis, treatment, and/or course of care. A total of 18 patients were able to avoid unnecessary surgery as a result of a PinnacleCare intervention.

The data demonstrates the potential for health advisory services and second opinions to optimize outcomes and avoid needless expense. One of the persistent challenges in health care today is access to expert physicians. With consumer directed health care plans, the value of health advisory services becomes even more evident as consumers struggle with vetting appropriate providers and treatment options for their complex conditions while seeking timely access to the care that they need. PinnacleCare is committed to providing objective, concierge-level support with the expert resources and access needed to help consumers tackle these complex challenges.

2015: *The DPC Journal* to release **its 2015 Annual Report and Market Trends Analyses** In The First Quarter of 2015

2015: *The DPC Journal* releases physician insight gathered in **a 2015 Industry Guidelines Proposal To Insurers and Legislators,** Second Quarter 2015

"The concierge model is a great option for physicians seeking more control over their time, their professional lives, and their ability to care for Patients. But it is by no means a financial cure-all. My life is so much better now.

It is a big improvement. I'm enjoying the benefit of more time for my family and my kids, more time to do administrative stuff during the workday rather than after-hours. But it is not like my financial woes suddenly disappeared, especially during the first year."

-Dr. D.
A Concierge Family Physician in CA

Great Expectations: What To Expect When You are Starting.

Over the past several years at *Concierge Medicine Today*, we have reported on a number of doctors who have struggled to find their place in the Concierge Medicine and DPC marketplace in the first two years. They have announced their new private-pay or retainer-based medicine practice service offerings and when they opened their doors they had some success. But about a year later, thirty percent of surveyed doctors interviewed were still unsure of their decision. We found that one in ten doctors in 2011 said they were worse off than before. What they will tell you is that no matter how hard you work, there are only 24 hours in a day and you have got to sleep during eight or nine of them.

The number one thing that causes these small businesses to fail is accounting and cash-flow problems. The second biggest thing is that they grow too quickly and fall in on themselves. Physicians and medical practice owners are sometimes scared to turn down any Patient at the start of entering into a Concierge Medicine or DPC medical practice. So they take everything that is offered, and things grow and grow and grow. The problem with that is it can become impossible to keep infrastructure, leadership, management and equipment in line with what you need to do the job right and keep the company running smoothly. That is why it is important to reach out to people who can help you.

Physicians and consultants in this industry will tell you that in the years following your transition to a Concierge Medicine or DPC model that it is critical to establish and set realistic expectations for the practice. A few of the expectations you should be aware of before you begin your journey into Concierge Medicine or implementing a DPC program in your practice are as follows:

1. **You Will Not Have As Many Patients As You Think ... For About 18-Months.**

Based upon the experience and interviews from hundreds of doctors over the years, we have found most Concierge and DPC doctors do not open with 600 or even 300 Patients right away. Choose a business model that works for you. Understand however, roughly 6 to 10% of your Patient base will eventually follow you into this new practice or enhanced access program. Consultants in the industry will conduct a feasibility assessment and set what they believe are achievable results for your practice based upon a number of factors. However, no one will make you promises they cannot keep. Meaning, if you have 3,000 Patients in your existing practice, you might want to expect you will have 300 Patients enrolled by the end of the membership enrollment period or by the end of the year.

2. **The Doctor Is The Best Sales Person.**

The reality is that most Concierge Medicine and DPC practices open below what they want and/or need to be financially successful in the first 18 months. Building Patient referrals, educating Patients about your services and continuing to build your "Know, Like and Trust Factor" with Patients is how your numbers will grow after the initial transition is over.

"It is difficult to be successful in Concierge Medicine without an established Patient base upon which knows, likes and trusts you." ~P.H., California

Furthermore, they must be willing to pay you for extended access and service beyond what insurance covers. The premise behind Concierge Medicine and most DPC medical offices is that doctors and Patients have the opportunity to spend more time one-on-one and building a closer, friendlier professional working relationship. The result of spending more time with your Patients, is that internal medicine and family doctors practicing in a concierge and DPC practice will ultimately have much smaller Patient panels than they would in the traditional managed care or insurance-based practice of fee for service (FFS) practice.

For The Medical Resident Or New Doctor ...

New Doctors motivated to move into this space and start a Concierge Medicine or DPC practice from the ground up with relatively little name recognition or Patient following, can expect slow growth. It is advised that you either: 1) find employment in the community and start your Concierge Medicine or DPC program on the side; 2) work at the local Urgent Care Clinic. Working at these types or clinics is moderately faster than hanging a shingle up on a building and sending out postcards with your name, fee and services on it. Urgent Care Clinic Patients typically have no primary care physician relationship. Most Urgent Care Clinics usually do not have a non-compete that they require their contracted physicians to sign – thus you might be able to establish primary care relationships with some Patients in this way. This is by far, the most desirable and fastest way to move into Concierge Medicine or the DPC space at a young age or in a community where you are virtually unknown.

Dr. Robert Nelson, who operates a successful DPC practice (www.mydocpps.com) while at the same time working for a local Urgent Care Clinic in the Atlanta area says, "The caveat here is that many Urgent Care facilities DO have non-compete clauses in their contracts that are specific for "urgent care" services. Be sure that you understand the details of any definition used for this term before you sign any such agreement. If you do launch your DPC or Concierge practice within the geographical area of the clinic that holds your non-compete agreement, make sure you do not advertise or use the non-compete terminology in your name or signage. For instance, if you offer Primary Care Services, that would not normally be seen as being in conflict with a non-compete agreement for urgent care services. Always have your attorney review all such issues before proceeding."

3. **History Shows An Average of 10% of Your Patients Will Enroll.**

A transition into this marketplace presents a number of challenges. One is holding onto as many current Patients as possible who have visited your practice over the past two years. History shows that an average of 10% of your Patients will eventually join your new subscription-based or membership program. The challenge beyond that is attracting and keeping new Patients.

"It is common for physicians, particularly those with long-standing Patients, to significantly underestimate 'ramp-up time' – how long it takes to get new people enrolled," said Helen Hadley, Founder and CEO of VantagePoint Healthcare Advisors in Hamden, CT.

4. Without Proper Planning, You Are Going To Be Cash-Strapped, At First.

Many of the Physicians, Business Administrators and Operators of these practices tell our news organizations, *The DPC Journal* and *Concierge Medicine Today*, that the first eighteen months are the toughest.

"Typically, there is a period after start-up when income goes way down as Patients decide whether to stay," said Allison McCarthy, a senior consultant in the northeast office of Corporate Health Group, a national consulting firm. "It often takes a good two years to bring the Patient level up to where it should be." At that point, physicians do better financially. In the interim, they are likely to struggle, particularly with those with large start-up costs, which can range from $50,000 to over $300,000.

5. Reach Out For Help.

If you think you can do this alone, think again. You need staff that supports you and believes in what your new practice model stands for, and, if married, a spouse that thinks you should do this and advice from a great accountant or two, a trusted attorney and a few savvy business people to help guide you along the way.

Specialists Considering Concierge Medicine Succeed When They Couple Their Care Specialty Services With Primary Care Services.

Specialists in Concierge Medicine, retainer medicine, DPC and boutique healthcare care account for approximately eight percent (8%) of the current concierge medical marketplace, according to *The Concierge Medicine Research Collective*. Specialists and primary care doctors alike are adding unique services to their practice encouraging more and more repeat visits with the Patient. Services and specialties include: cardiology; pediatrics; OB/GYN; neurology; hormone replacement therapy, anti-aging solutions and more.

Attracted to the opportunity to provide concierge medicine's hallmark model of personalized care, physicians in subspecialties such as cardiology, endocrinology, pulmonology, and others are increasingly converting their practices, and reporting increased professional and personal satisfaction, according to Michael Friedlander, Principal at national healthcare consulting firm Specialdocs.

One such example recently reported on by *Concierge Medicine Today* had to do with an OB/GYN physician in the southeast. She understood that each of her Patients had a primary care doctor (PCP) that is chosen from their desired insurance provider's list. But many of the tests she was ordering were the same as the PCP. Because a Patient's medical information and history is not shared between various Medical Providers unless specifically obtained by the Patient's physician or provided by the Patient themselves, there is currently little collaboration or synchronization between medical providers. A Patient must try to provide each new Doctor their prior healthcare history explaining what prior Medical Providers have tested and diagnosed. The OB/GYN found this lack of information and duplicate tests and procedures frustrating for many of her Patients. So, she decided to update her internal medicine boards so she could provide primary care services as part of her Concierge Medicine practice.

Duplicate tests and procedures are time consuming and costly. The methodology does not constitute effective and efficient medical care. Expanding your service to include Primary Care can be a good solution.

Leading cardiologist John R. Levinson, MD, PhD, founder of the country's first concierge subspecialty practice, AllCare Medical, LLC, in Boston, says: "Those specialties where patients have a longitudinal relationship with their doctor to work on chronic problems are an ideal fit for the concierge model. If you're the kind of cardiologist who helps patients work on chronic valve disease, coronary disease, or other areas of preventive cardiology, a concierge practice vastly improves your ability to provide the very best care for each and every patient."

Agrees E. Thomas Arne, Jr., DO, FACC, who transitioned his cardiology practice to the concierge model last spring with the help of Specialdocs: "So many risk factors circle around heart health—diabetes, high blood pressure, high cholesterol—that being able to assume the primary care role and manage these issues upfront makes cardiology an ideal fit for concierge medicine." The opportunity to treat the whole patient and address their entire scope of medical issues translates to better, more personalized medicine, according to Dr. Arne.

Top 5 Complaints Heard About Concierge Medicine.

While most concierge medical practices maintain a very high Patient retention average of approximately 92%-94%*. It is important to tell you what we hear from Patients reading our stories, news articles and those looking for doctors accepting new Patients in their area. *Source: *Concierge Medicine Today*, March 2010-2013)

When we recently analyzed over 1,000 prospective Concierge Medicine Patient search requests obtained over several months on our site (www.ConciergeMedicineToday.com) — **nearly 30% of Patients are leaving one Concierge Doctor and seeking another.** What is wrong with this picture? The retention rate is high, but what is happening to those that are leaving and more importantly, why are they leaving your practice?

So, we asked them the question 'What, if anything, could be improved or would you change regarding your previous concierge/direct medical practice?' The findings may surprise you. We have listed them in order of importance according to the Patient responses. They include:

 # 1) Rude Office Manager And/or Staff.

In some cases, physicians employ their wives as front office staff. In most practices, this is great. However, in some practices, when the Patient knows that it is the doctor's wife that is being curt or ill-tempered, the Patient is much more reluctant to tell the physician about their experience. In other cases, the physician has employed his/her front office staff for many years and is aware of the problem but unwilling to make a change because of emotion, history, misplaced loyalty or finances.

2) Person Scheduling Appointment(s) Is Ill-Tempered And Seems Annoyed...More Than Two Times In A Row.

The first time might be acceptable. But if it happens again, the Patient starts rethinking their decision, the leadership of the physician and their membership in the practice entirely. Every day, people turn to friends and colleagues for recommendations regarding services, especially healthcare services. Because word-of-mouth referrals are free, you cannot beat the return on investment. If the person who is scheduling your appointments is not friendly, inviting, warm or knowledgeable, you should correct this person(s) quickly or consider a replacement.

A True Story.

A physician in the suburbs of Atlanta, GA recently let his unfriendly Office Manager go and hired a friendly person to fill this position. The Office Manager recently told CMT how many negative comments they receive about the former Office Manager and how this change made a big difference. They also stated that the physician is receiving verbal praise about once a day for their new hire from current Patients. Former Patient appointments are also picking up dramatically at the practice.

3) Over-Promised And Under-Served + Appointment Scheduling Was Not Any Easier.

The rule to remember here, do not promise more than you can deliver. In 2012, this was the number one reason why Patients were searching for another concierge physician, according to Patient surveys received by *Concierge Medicine Today's* physician search engine, *DOC FINDER*. This complaint dropped to third on the list of complaints in 2013. An improvement, but still, something about which Patients are concerned.

One former Patient of a retainer-based physician in Florida told us that they paid for their annual membership fee for the entire year. Upon calling to schedule their first appointment, they were put on hold for 19 minutes. The appointment calendar was full and she could not get into see her physician for three weeks. Three weeks later when she arrived at the practice, the waiting room was full. Nothing about the new business model or practice seemed to have changed whatsoever. When her name was called, she was visited in the exam room by the Nurse Practitioner, not the physician she paid and/or signed up to see. 'This was not in the brochure...'

4) Economic Conditions of Households Under $100k (Combined)

In a concierge medical practice you are marketing a relationship-based service product which is essentially accessed for a fee. It is a specialized, personal and relationship-based service that not everyone knows is affordable — but it is beginning to catch on.

5) Patients(s) Did Not Use The Membership As Much As They Thought.

This was particularly common in households with a combined income between $100k-$150k/year. Be that as it may, we are not suggesting any price change to adapt to underutilizing patients at this time. *Concierge Medicine Today* does believe practices gain a competitive value advantage when the following Value-Added Services are provided without changing your annual fee. Patients will perceive that they are receiving additional value at no additional cost, which will encourage them to continue their relationship with you. Considering incorporating these ideas into your practice on a weekly, if not daily routine:

- Hand Written Cards: i.e. Thank You; Thanksgiving; Christmas; Birthday; Valentine's Day; Veteran's Day; Bereavement Card(s), etc.
- Cost Reduction Specials on Tangible Items
- Texting Availability Directly To The Physician's Cell Phone
- Text Message Appointment Reminders
- Access To Safe, Secure, Online Interactive Medical ID Bracelet; Wrist Band; Tag; Shoe ID; Ankle ID or Executive ID Bracelet

Here's A Piece Of Advice Some Savvy And Highly Successful Doctors Will Tell You.

If you already have great employees, make sure they understand what you are trying to do with your new practice. Education and mental buy-in amongst your staff is key. If they do not believe in what you are about to do, you may need to make some tough decisions. If you are a one-person show in your medical office right now, you can reach out to a few friends and family members to help you or, if they do not have the skills you need, you should connect with a quality Concierge Medicine or DPC conversion consultant that can help you.

There are so many to choose from these days. From individuals experienced with your kind of needs to more franchised models that have proven track records and a long history of success.

It is commonly assumed that doctors who enter "Concierge Medicine"
are driven to do so by money. What most doctors who have been there and
done that will tell you is ... 'I'm fueled by a passion to help my Patients.
I am now allowed the opportunity to problem-solve and make life a little easier, better and
cheaper for my Patients.'

~Concierge Medicine Today, © 2014

Physician Benefits

"I became a concierge physician for the same reason I became a doctor – I want to help people. With this model, I can continue to help people even when traditional medicine changes significantly. When a patient has a "one more thing, Doctor...," the last thing I want to do is to cut the patient off. Patients deserve to be involved in their care and receive the valuable service of planning for optimal health with the guidance of a family physician who is dedicated to the care of the patient." ~Dr. Brian Nadolne, MD, Marietta, GA

How Will Transforming Into A DPC Practice Affect My Patients?

Generally, Concierge Medicine and most DPC physicians have a panel of between 600 and 800 Patients. In typical FFS settings, the Patient panels tend to range from between 2,000 and 5,000 per internal medicine family physician. This often results in Patients losing relationship and regular access to a physician if they elect not to participate in a Concierge Medicine or DPC relationship.

Patients who receive personal care in the Concierge Medicine or DPC practice will find their experience and healthcare services significantly different when compared with the care and experience they receive in traditional primary care, insurance-based, managed care practice setting, and primarily spending increased time with their doctor.

There are a number of reported outcomes of increasing visit time, including improved Patient experience of care, and improved clinical outcomes as Patients become more engaged with their doctor and begin to take an active role in their own health care under the direction of their Concierge Doctor.

What Is Expected of Me and My Time?

Patients inside Concierge Medicine and/or DPC practices find it much easier to access their physicians and the practice offices.

A number of practices now offer:
- E-Consultations;
- iPhone Facetime Visits;
- Online Prescription Renewals;
- Skype Visits
- Annual Physical
- House Calls
- After-Hours Consults
- Prescription Questions And Call-Ins
- More In-Depth And Researched Treatment Options
- On-Time Appointments
- Friendly Staff Who Know Each Patients First Name
- Specialist Coordination

- Lab And Testing Discounts And More.

Additionally, many of these practices have expanded their operating hours while opening scheduling for same-day visits. Most, if not all, Concierge Medicine practices provide Patients a way to contact their doctor 24 hours a day so as to avoid inconvenient and costly hospitalizations.

By Implementing A Concierge Medicine Style Business Model Physicians Are Able To:

- Earn a predictable salary.
- Spend more time with your Patients.
- Enjoy a Less stressful working environment.
- Reduce administrative burden on office staff.
- Retain between 85%-97% of your "enrolled/signed-up" Patients each year with very little effort.
- Typically enjoy annual growth between 1% to 7% through Patient referrals, online marketing, local press and media exposure, etc.
- Typically offer 24/7 access to the doctor, same day appointments, longer appointment times and a greater degree of personalized attention to their Patients.
- Spend between 30 - 60 minutes with each Patient.
- Reduce the total amount of medication their Patients intake by 50-95%, according to surveys obtained from concierge/direct care physicians operating in the concierge medical movement in the U.S.
- Have less intrusion from the everyday burdens brought on by managed care, insurance and administrative headaches.
- Employ between 1-2.5 employees (59%); 3-5 employees (32%)
- Lower elective, non-elective, emergent, urgent, avoidable and unavoidable hospital admissions. This was demonstrated among the MDVIP members compared to non-members for the years 2006, 2007, 2008, 2009 and 2010, demonstrating consistent reductions – Source: December 2012 issue of *The American Journal of Managed Care*;
- Create a profitable, irresistible and predictable practice environment that you, your Patients and staff can enjoy.
- Focus your time and energy on practicing medicine, not business operations.

Facts About Concierge Medicine and DPC Practices:

- In a May 2014 *Medscape* interview, *Concierge Medicine Today* and *The DPC Journal*, said that the current marketplace supports a total of 12,000 physicians operating in a free market delivery model – whether by Concierge Medicine or a DPC business model across the U.S. Digging deeper, they find that there are slightly more than 4000 physicians "who are verifiably, actively practicing concierge medicine or DPC across the United States, with probably another 8000 practicing under the radar."
- Concierge physicians generally have between 100 and 1,000 Patients, a much lower number compared with the usual panel of 2,000-3,000 Patients in insurance-based practices. Fees vary widely, from $600 to $5,000 per Patient per year.
- Over 66% of current U.S. concierge physicians operating practices today are internal medicine specialists.
- The second most popular medical specialty in Concierge Medicine is family practice;
- Surprisingly there are an increasing number of concierge cardiology, dental and pediatric DPC practices arising since February of 2009.
- Female concierge physician practices generally fill up faster than their male counterparts primarily due to the target audience of females. Those Moms serve as the healthcare CEO of the family.
- The average age of a concierge physician is between 50-59 (46%); age 40-49 (30%); age 30-39 (14%); age 60-69 (8%); age 70+ (1-2%).
- After converting to a Concierge Medicine practice, doctors changed the following in their office space: reduced the total amount of leased space; updated or added new signage; reduced staff; painted and redecorated lobby, hallways, exam rooms and changed furniture; added a self-serve single cup coffee and tea station in their lobby; extended office hours one to two days per week to accommodate early morning and evening hour visits; added a flat screen television to the lobby. Note: less than 6% of doctors found they needed to move from their existing practice to a new location.
- Doctors entering the Concierge Medicine model paid for their transition largely by investing personal assets (i.e. savings, 401k, etc.). Others found that working slowly towards the transition and funding the expenses necessary to transition were best acquired through picking up extra shifts at a local Urgent Care or ER. Few doctors (approx. 13%) found traditional lending methods through banks to be the most beneficial way to pay for the expenses necessary to transition into Concierge Medicine.
- Franchise and consulting fees can move from five-figures and easily into the six figures. According to *Concierge Medicine Today*, the average cost is between $150,000 – $250,000 over a period of two to five years and in some rare cases, even longer. Some consultants have quoted figures less than $60,000. So there is a significant range dependent upon what you want the Consultant to do. Dependent upon your practice, it is demographics, your bedside manner, Patient surveys (very important), complexity of internal operations, financial feasibility analysis, and many other variables, a Concierge Medicine or DPC practice may or may not be the right option for you.
- Figures in the past from MDVIP stories and articles cite Patient retention is between 95% and 98% each year.

- In late 2012, a report from MDVIP and the peer-reviewed, American Journal of Managed Care, stated that Patients under the care of MDVIP-affiliated primary care physicians experience a dramatic decrease in hospitalizations versus comparable non-MDVIP Patients, This was the first published study done on hospital utilization in the MDVIP personalized healthcare model found a 79% reduction in hospital admissions for Medicare Patients, and a 72% decrease for those with commercial insurance between the ages of 35-64 in MDVIP-affiliated practices. As a result, MDVIP, the most prominent national network of primary care physicians, delivered a one-year savings in excess of $300 million.
- The study also found decreased MDVIP hospital readmission rates for Medicare members when compared to the 2009 readmission rates for non-MDVIP Medicare Patients, for such conditions as acute MI (heart attack), CHF (congestive heart failure) and pneumonia. MDVIP readmission rates are below 2% for these conditions compared to the national averages that range from a low of 16% to a high of 24%.

"*Despite what we hear in the media about the increase in concierge and private-pay physicians growing across America, there are simply not enough of these [Concierge Medicine, direct care or membership medicine-style] physicians in the U.S. to meet the current demand,*"
says an HR Manager based in
Atlanta, Georgia.

The Ethical Dilemmas

"Concierge Medicine must be treated seriously by physicians and Patients alike because it is a concept that is here to stay. Paying a set annual fee for "special services" may appear to some to focus on money and greed but to others it may be redirecting the focus of medicine back to preventing disease and seeking wellness. If concierge physicians are successful in preventing illness and keeping Patients healthier then it is in the best interest of Patients, physicians and society as a whole." ~Peter A. Clark SJ, PhD Professor of Medical Ethics and Director, Institute of Catholic Bioethics, Saint Joseph's University

There are a wide variety of philosophical opinions that about the ethics of Concierge Medicine. The Internet has become a canvas of thoughts for many to express their views, both for and against, on the topic. We have seen and heard everything from 'concierge care' only worsens the doctor shortage to 'it is elitist and serves only the wealthy in America' to 'I thought doctors were supposed to do no harm.'

While many of these ideologies circulate around a personal philosophical and political viewpoint, that is not the purpose of this section or even this book. What we are here to do is briefly highlight for you the common issues that your colleagues, business leaders, insurers, friends and even those around you might have and how you can educate yourself to respond. The main ethical issues you have probably encountered, or possibly even wrestled with yourself, focus on: whether Concierge Medicine will result in a two-tiered medical system based upon economics; add to the already increasing doctor shortage; is this a form of Patient abandonment?; and how does this new form of medical practice address the belief that doctors have a professional obligation to provide care for all those in need, especially the most vulnerable of Patients?

C.J. Miles, MBAHCM, MSA Research Analyst at the AMAC Foundation writes ... 'Any type of healthcare and health insurance-related issue is going to have legal and ethical issues that everyone will not agree on. The bottom line with concierge medicine is that it is quickly growing, presumably due to physicians and patients fed up with the current state of America's healthcare system and where it could be going due to The Affordable Care Act. In fact, even with the growing number of concierge physicians, "the number of patients who are seeking concierge medical care in the past 24 months is far greater than the actual number of primary care and family practice concierge physicians available to service them" (Concierge Medicine Today; CMT, 2014b, para. 22). Only time will tell how this will pan out, but for now, it looks like this is where our country is heading.'

Will Concierge Medicine Worsen The Shortage Of Primary Care Doctors?

Simply answered, no.

The numbers do not match-up to media touted reports. Though it is true that most Concierge Doctors decrease the size of their existing practices when they switch to a DPC business model, there is already a mass exodus of doctors to this model from primary care and family medicine. *Concierge Medicine Today*, released a statement late in 2013 stating that They have found that the number of Patients who are seeking these types of Concierge Medicine and DPC healthcare practitioners is far greater than the actual number of "concierge" primary care and DPC family practice doctors available to serve them.

Furthermore, *The Concierge Medicine Research Collective* reports that it is extremely difficult to find a Concierge Medicine or DPC physician in rural areas such as: Idaho; North Dakota; South Dakota; Louisiana; Mississippi and others. Oftentimes, less than half-a-dozen practitioners serve an entire state.

In 2013 a national survey of physicians that Merritt Hawkins completed on behalf of The Physicians Foundation shed some light on this question. The survey garnered responses from some 14,000 physicians, who revealed a wide range of information regarding their morale, practice metrics and practice plans. Physicians were asked what changes they plan to make in their practices over the next one to three years. Close to seven percent of physicians responding indicated they plan to switch to a concierge practice.

Now, let's look at the math. Most people do not understand or are aware that nearly 80% of the Concierge Medicine doctors' offices and 40% of DPC Clinics operating today across the U.S. treat on average, 600 Patients but that many of these also have an insurance side [approx. 1,900 Patients on avg.] to their practice. Meaning, most Concierge Doctors accept and continue to participate in their HMO, PPO and managed care insurance contracts long after they have announced to a local community that they now offer a Concierge Medicine membership program to allow "more access to your doctor."

Where Patient abandonment discussions along with moral and ethical issues, typically arise is when the doctor discontinues all insurance relationships in his/her practice and simply charges a cash fee for his/her services, thereby releasing 1,900 Patients from the practice.

Understanding the insured component of a true Concierge Medicine practice, 2,500 Patients do not typically leave the practice because a doctor isn't able to treat them or keep them as part of his/her panel. Conservatively estimating that most traditional [non-concierge] primary care and family physicians have a Patient panel of 2,500 Patients, let's say 6.9% of 13,575 doctors convert to Concierge Medicine. This equates to about 950 doctors out of 13,575 transitioning their business model to Concierge Medicine. Thereby leaving 13,050 doctors to serve a population of roughly the same amount of insured Patients.

So, where is the shortage? If research says only 15% of Concierge Doctors do not participate in insurance that means that 15% of 950 doctors will provide cash-only services to a Patient base of roughly 600 Patients each. Backing into the math, that means 143 [15% of 950 doctors] doctors will treat about 600 Patients each equating to a serviced Patient population of 85,800 [143 x 600]. If each of the 143 doctors had 2,500 Patients that means 271,700 Patients no longer have a doctor that will accept insurance. Divide this Patient population number [271,700] by the amount of doctors left who are still accepting insurance and choose to not participate in a Concierge Medicine practice whatsoever [13,050], that means each of the 13,050 doctors' offices have the opportunity to welcome about 20 new Patients into their practice. *(Source: Concierge Medicine Today, 2013, Michael Tetreault, Editor)*

What the Merritt Hawkins data also states is ... *it is interesting to note here that physician practice "owners" are more likely to embrace Concierge Medicine than other types of physicians, presumably because they have an entrepreneurial mindset.*

It is also important to mention here that there are a lot of conflicting numbers about the growth each year of Concierge Medicine and private-pay healthcare offices touted by industry sources and media outlets. To date, key physician leaders in the industry tell us that most crucial data compiled about this industry's growth has come from The Merritt Hawkins Study, MDVIP and thru *Concierge Medicine Today's* research arm, *The Concierge Medicine Research Collective.*

"Obamacare helped," writes Sonja Horner, President at Private Medical Partners in an editorial contribution published in *Concierge Medicine Today,* October 2014. "I know, trust me it's hard to admit, but I'm referencing how it helped consumers understand the sheer demand for the small number of physicians in this country compared to the growing number of people that need care. It also caused the media, in all forms, to cover options to Obamacare and concierge medical care was one of those options. *USA Today* and *Forbes* did a beautiful job of educating consumers through info-graphics about concierge medicine and even so far as to recommend it in an article on, "How to Survive Obamacare?"."

While the argument that Concierge Medicine will exacerbate the doctor shortage is continuing, we can now see that there is actually a proven, viable history that these types of healthcare practitioners are showing that primary care can be saved. This argument will keep the media and nay-sayers busy for the next couple of years but the marketplace consumer is the one who is showing all of us that we are a long way from seeing a Concierge Doctor in every neighborhood, but we need them and, we need more of them.

"Young doctors are refusing to go into primary care medicine," notes Dr. Steven Knope of Tucson, Arizona in his writings about The Myths of Concierge Medicine. "This is due to the fact that practicing primary care medicine in our current broken system, seeing 30 Patients per day, making only one-third to one-fourth of what a specialist makes, have created an understandable shortage of doctors willing to practice primary care medicine. Over the long run, the only way to increase the number of qualified primary care doctors is to make the profession more attractive, both from a professional and financial perspective. It is our current broken system that has caused a shortage of primary care doctors; and if we stay on the old path, it will only get worse."

"I didn't become a doctor to bankrupt my Patients..."
~Dr. Jordan Grumet

Is Concierge Medicine Elitist?

According to *Concierge Medicine Today*, executives and celebrities account for less than 4% of Patients searching for this type of care. So, despite the high-powered executives using Concierge Medicine, executives of all ages and backgrounds are not the most popular Patient demographic searching for concierge medical doctors across America today.

Additionally, *The Concierge Medicine Research Collective*, published an August 2010 to February 2013 summary of online polling and survey results received from Patients of Concierge Medicine which revealed that top-level executives account for less than 6% of the Patients searching for this type of healthcare.

"Consumers buy what they understand," writes Sonja Horner in a *Concierge Medicine Today* editorial. "It has taken years for the industry to educate consumers about the basic components of concierge medicine. Build upon that existing knowledge base and take the time to further educate them on how your practice uses labs, technology and other tools that will elevate their health. Thanks to industry pioneers like MDVIP there are published studies that show that their members experience a reduction in hospitalizations by just over 70%. You may not like to reference a competitor like MDVIP, but as a starting point your practice can harness this study to further demonstrate value."

We thought that the numbers would be higher given the media's love affair with touting Concierge Medicine's elitist stereotype. Add to that the number of consultants in the industry stating that Concierge Doctors should gear their marketing efforts towards executives and that a significant number of practices are comprised of this clientele, most successful Concierge Doctors will tell you that the obvious conclusion to this myth is that a wealthy audience is not necessarily the primary subscriber to this type of healthcare.

So, if it is not the wealthy, celebrity-type or high-level executives who are searching for this type of care, who is looking for Concierge Medicine?

To find the answer to this question, we turned to our national concierge physician search engine, *DOC FINDER*, at www.ConciergeMedicineToday.com. It receives daily requests from prospective and first-time Patients as well as current concierge Patients looking to make a change to another Concierge Medicine or DPC provider. We found:

- 49% of all concierge physician searches by Patients are for an Individual.
- 23% of all concierge physician searches are for Couples, with no children.
- 21% of all concierge physician searches are for Families, with children.
- 4% of all concierge physician searches received are for Business Owners/Top Executives.
- 3% Allowable Margin of Error +/- 3%.

The information found here provides evidence that Concierge Medicine is not just for the deep-pocketed celebrity, sports star or high-powered executive. In fact, over 50% of Concierge Medicine Patients make a combined household income of less than $100,000 per year.

This data should be very encouraging to the public, as well as the media and practicing Concierge Medicine and DPC doctor community. A concept, initially thought of by many as healthcare for the rich, is now accessible and affordable for families, couples with and without children, individuals, seniors, young families and people who cannot afford the high cost of health insurance.

Legal experts and business leaders favor the concept of Concierge Medicine, but with the proper guidelines and safeguards in place. Most believe that Concierge Medicine is a desirable, affordable and beneficial option for Patients, physicians, and good for society.

While most people, once they understand how Concierge Medicine works and the advantage to their pocketbooks are in favor of this type of Patient-physician relationship. However, also recognized is the need for development of specific guidelines; formalized franchise standards; professional standards; recommendations for these physicians. For example, in 2003, The American Medical Association issued boutique care (i.e. Concierge Medicine and DPC) guidelines.

In 2012, The American Academy of Family Practice (AAFP) formally stated their positive opinion about Concierge Medicine's companion model, DPC. In February of 2014, the American College of Private Physicians (ACPP) formed in the marketplace in an effort to focus on credentialing doctors, advocacy to employers, unions, government and the like to benefit industry nationwide. Additionally, another formal practice certification in private medicine was announced by the American Academy of Private Physicians (AAPP) at the Fall Summit in Miami, Florida on October 10-11, 2014. The AAPP will now endorse standards of care and compliance credentialing.

"This certification is first of its kind" according to AAPP president Matthew Priddy, M.D. "This process will enable private medicine and DPC physicians to certify their practice is compliant with both state and federal regulations."

There are significant ethical questions surrounding Concierge Medicine. Elitist healthcare obviously being the most popular. However, to critics of Concierge Medicine, you will also hear discussions about the ethical treatment of Patients and 'do no harm.' Does Concierge Medicine add to the primary care shortage? These are valid questions and thoughts that need to discussed in local doctors' offices and with the health insurance leadership managing large insurance programs. For the purpose of this book, we are highlighting some of the most common questions raised about this type of healthcare. We believe it is up to you and your Patients to have these discussions and come to your own conclusions about the efficacy and ethics of Concierge Medicine, DPC healthcare and retail medicine style doctors' offices.

"*Growth in any service industry, particularly healthcare depends largely on consumer spending. Concierge Medicine and its familial companion, DPC are approaching a tipping point.*" *says Michael Tetreault, Executive Director of The Collective and Editor of the industry's trade publications, Concierge Medicine Today and The DPC Journal.* "*Doctors are now deciding between what they have to do and what they want to do.*"

"*We believe it is up to you and your Patients to decide and come to your own conclusions about the efficacy and ethics of Concierge Medicine, DPC healthcare and retail medicine style doctors' offices.*"

~Catherine Sykes, Publisher of The DPC Journal and Concierge Medicine Today, Speaker

Salary Expectations

Despite the widespread economic downturn of the last 4-5 years, membership in concierge practices continues to grow. Annual renewal rates have stayed consistently between 85%-95%. The Concierge Medicine and DPC business model of primary care practice is growing at a brisk 10-12% annual pace nationwide, now over 12,000+ practices across the U.S. according to *The Concierge Medicine Research Collective* in an interview with *Medscape*, May of 2014. It also appears to be fairly recession-proof. Moreover, it can significantly improve clinical outcomes for Patients, even those of fairly modest means.

We release regular summaries and findings of data highlighting Concierge Medicine physician salaries. The data was based upon surveys, polling analysis and verbal interviews and feedback received from the concierge physician community across the U.S. from 2009 to 2012. Here are some of the highlights:

- The top 4 most popular specialties in Concierge Medicine are: primary care; family medicine; cardiology and pediatrics.
- The majority of Concierge Doctors (approximately 25%) earn between $200,000 – $300,000 per year.
- On average, a Concierge Doctor earns relatively the same salary of a specialist, such as a radiologist or cardiologist.
- Most Concierge physicians do a significant amount of charity work, often seeing about 5 to 11 percent of their Patients free-of-charge.
- Concierge Medicine puts the incomes of internists and family practitioners on the same earning level with their colleagues.
- For the past five years, four states across the U.S. continue to have a significant amount of Concierge Doctors providing concierge medical care: Florida; California; Pennsylvania and Virginia. All of these states continue have a significant number of people (most over age 50) seeking out Concierge Medicine and DPC doctors.
- The most common age of Concierge Doctor is between 40-59 years of age.
- Most Concierge Doctors and DPC physicians treat six to eight Patients per day.
- Female Concierge Doctors fill up their concierge practices 30% faster than men.

2013 Concierge Medicine Physician Compensation Data

- 14% of Concierge Doctors earn $1 – $100,000 per year.
- 23% of Concierge Doctors earn $100,000 – $200,000 per year.
- 25% of Concierge Doctors earn $200,000 – $300,000 per year.
- 21% of Concierge Doctors earn $300,000 – $400,000 per year.
- 6% of Concierge Doctors earn $400,000 – $500,000 per year.
- 7% of Concierge Doctors earn $500,000 – $600,000 per year.
- 1% of Concierge Doctors earn $600,000 – $700,000 per year.
- 3% of Concierge Doctors earn $700,000 per year and up.

Today's Hospitalist conducted their own limited survey of non-concierge hospitalist physicians and found that when compared to traditional, insurance-based physicians working in a hospital setting, the salary ranges very widely with some hospitalists making between $150,000 to $227,000 in annual income.

2013 Concierge Medicine Physician Compensation Data
Source: *The Concierge Medicine Research Collective*, ConciergeMedicineToday.com

- 13% of concierge physicians reported a decrease in income.
- 25% of concierge physicians reported income remained the same.
  62% of concierge physicians reported an increase in income.

In a 2013 MedScape Survey, they found that Concierge Medicine and DPC practices are on the rise, albeit a slow one. Doctors joining ACOs jumped up from 3% to 16%.

Overall, Concierge Medicine is thriving in metropolitan markets. Most, with the majority of physician incomes remaining the same or increasing slightly. Career satisfaction with the given field also remains high. According to *Concierge Medicine Today*, only 18% of physicians stated they would not make the same decision again. In previous years, it was 25% but even so, the number overall is low and satisfaction with the business model is high when compared to traditional, insurance-based or managed care medical practices.

2014 Concierge Medicine Physician Compensation Data
Source: *The Concierge Medicine Research Collective*, ConciergeMedicineToday.com

Concierge Medicine Today released data in May of 2014 summarizing Concierge Medicine and DPC physician salaries in the U.S. The data is based upon surveys, polling analysis and verbal responses received from concierge doctors throughout the U.S. during the 2013-2014 calendar years. Here are some of the highlights:

- 49% of Concierge Physicians reported that their annual salary/earnings in 2013 increased compared to years past.
- 41% of Concierge Physicians reported that their annual salary/earnings in 2013 decreased compared to years past.
- 10% of Concierge Physicians reported that their annual salary/earnings in 2013 remained unchanged or the same compared to years past.
- Reasons given by Concierge Physicians for decreases in salary included: increasing business taxes (both State and Federal) and fewer patients were renewing their membership with the practice.

Some physicians are becoming concierge doctors within the hospital environment to both reduce administrative time and earn more income. Still others are choosing to maintain solo concierge medicine practices, approximately 85%, according to three years of physician polling data conducted by *The Concierge Medicine Research Collective*.

On average, a Concierge Physician earns the equivalent salary of a specialist, such as a cardiologist or a radiologist. Most concierge doctors do a significant amount of charity work, often seeing about 10 percent of their patient's free-of-charge or at a reduced fee. Concierge Medicine puts the incomes of internists and family practitioners on par with their colleagues. A 2012 Medscape study found that the average salary for a primary care physician ranged from $156,000 to $315,000, while *Bloomberg Businessweek* reported that the average salary for a Concierge Physician ranged from $150,000 to $300,000.

Concierge Medicine Physician Compensation Data from 2013-2014

- 14% of Concierge Physicians earn $1 – $100,000 per year.
- 31% of Concierge Physicians earn $100,000 – $200,000 per year.
- 19% of Concierge Physicians earn $200,000 – $300,000 per year.
- 14% of concierge Physicians earn $300,000 – $400,000 per year.
- 13% of Concierge Physicians earn $400,000 – $1 Million per year.
- 9% of Concierge Physicians earn $1 Million per year and above.

Concierge Physicians within the hospital environment may enjoy the best of both worlds. They see a reduced number of patients on a day-to-day basis while earning higher salaries and handling less administrative obligations than they would in a traditional private practice setting. When compared to traditional, insurance-based physicians working in a hospital setting, Today's Hospitalist conducted their own limited survey of non-concierge Hospitalist physicians and found that the salary ranges very widely with some Hospitalists making between $150,000 to $227,000 in annual income.

Concierge Medicine Physician Compensation Data from 2012-2013

- 14% of Concierge Physicians earned $1 – $100,000 per year.
- 23% of Concierge Physicians earned $100,000 – $200,000 per year.
- 25% of Concierge Physicians earned $200,000 – $300,000 per year.
- 21% of Concierge Physicians earned $300,000 – $400,000 per year.
- 17% of Concierge Physicians earned $400,000 – $1 Million per year and above.

In some instances, a concierge medicine office will serve 600 patients and these membership fees can generate a gross income of $900,000 (600 patients x $1,500). If the practice bills the patient's insurance for additional healthcare services, these insurance reimbursements will also add to the gross income of a concierge medical practice. One physician told Medical Economics recently that membership fees in his practice account for two-thirds of his gross revenue, while insurance revenue brings in the remainder. Many physicians in this industry report that switching from a traditional, insurance based, managed care style medical practice business model to a membership-based, direct-pay business model helps reduce administrative costs, operational expenditures and staffing. With a reduced patient load from that of a traditional primary care practice, concierge medicine and cash-only clinics are more about improving the patient-physician relationship, eliminating costly distractions from a medical practice, such as insurance filings, and about simplifying the doctor-patient relationship based on price transparency. Many are now offering extended hours that cater to a more patient-centered relationship with a physician.

The National Landscape.

From 1996 to 2014, *Concierge Medicine Today* estimates Concierge Medicine and DPC physician's number approximately 12,000+ physicians and/or physician clinics across the U.S. This is according to in-depth review and examination of the marketplace and interviews with various corporate industry leaders with national perspectives and holdings.

It is important to note, *The Concierge Medicine Research Collective* and *Concierge Medicine Today*, work hand-in-hand to search for concierge physicians who currently practice and operate their practice(s) in a Concierge Medicine business practice model. To accomplish this, we conduct exhaustive online research and utilize: search results; phone calls; directories; surveys; business affiliations and address maps to locate and maintain accurate numbers of Concierge Medicine physicians throughout the U.S. Our goal is to accurately track the current number of physicians and provide relevant educational information and data to interested parties and stakeholders requesting information about this emerging and dynamic medical industry.

As it pertains to discrepancies between the figures quoted by various organizations, we would conclude that while our numbers vary from other organizations, other figures may also have validity. Our figures do not include those doctors that practice "below the radar". Meaning, they have practices that may not be advertised as or necessarily considered true concierge medical business models. However, they may provide some form(s) of service(s) in their practice that is similar to these medical practice models. There are also doctors who are practicing in a concierge practice model but their practices are "closed" or "limited" and are not accepting new Patients. They are usually growing via Patient referrals. These doctors may not be included in our research as these doctors oftentimes do no advertising or public communications conveying their practice model information.

We have also found that the states which appear to be the leanest from a concierge medical service population perspective include the States of: Hawaii; Idaho; Iowa; Mississippi; Maine; New Hampshire and South Dakota.

What you might be surprised about is that the number of Patients who are seeking concierge medical care and DPC doctors is far greater than the actual number of primary care and family practice doctors available to serve them. Concierge medical and DPC offices in rural areas like Idaho; North Dakota; South Dakota; Alaska; Hawaii; Louisiana; and Mississippi are in short supply. Oftentimes, we are learning that there are less than half-a-dozen practitioners to serve an entire state.

"*Although national media has reported increasing numbers of concierge, private-pay physicians in America, there are still not enough Concierge Medicine physicians to meet current consumer demand.*

According to Michael Tetreault, Editor of Concierge Medicine Today, search activity on his magazine's Concierge Medicine, DPC doctors' search engine has increased tremendously since the 2012 election and throughout January 2013. Even if you include all of the doctors who claim to be DPC or operate a Concierge Medicine practice, the supply still falls short.

Source: http://www.practicebuilders.com/blog/healthcare-news/demand-for-concierge-medicine-outpacing-supply-part-1-of-2/#sthash.pkNS3sIR.dpuf

New York Usually Sets The Trend For the Country.
NYC Sees Dramatic Growth In Concierge Medicine From 2008-2014

Concierge Medicine Today reported that the State of New York and more specifically, the City of New York, has experienced a significant increase in the number of Concierge Medicine doctors, DPC physician clinics and private-pay primary care practices in the past 5 years.

In 2008, there were approximately 28 "verified" Concierge Medicine doctors practicing and treating Patients in the New York, NY metro area. Today, we have found that there are over 124 Concierge Medicine doctors treating Patients in the same metro area of New York City.

In recent years, significant venture capital has been poured into the Concierge Medicine and DPC marketplace. Investment groups are not only attracted to these transparent and innovative healthcare clinics but they see them as a viable investment for their clients. Where Concierge Medicine and DPC practices are struggling is in the ability to scale their business for mass-market and employer appeal.

The future looks bright for those doctors considering a career in cash-only or retainer medicine. Large groups like MedLion, MDVIP, Qliance and One Medical are building and scaling successful medical practices across the country and in various parts of their home states. These are attractive to investors like: Cambia Health (a large Blue Shield company); Google Ventures; Proctor and Gamble; Benchmark Capital; DAG Ventures; Oak Investment Partners: Maverick Capital and others.

More recently, *Entrepreneur Magazine, Forbes* and others published their list of The Best States for Entrepreneurs. Analyzing that data along with data compiled from over 5,000+ small businesses and Concierge Medicine consumers, *Concierge Medicine Today* identified a list of The Best Cities and States for a Career in Concierge Medicine and DPC in 2013-2014. The cities and states on this list support not only small business but healthcare innovation. They provide a growing but friendly Patient population who support these types of modern medical delivery systems.

"Direct practices should be successful in most cities and states where there is an inadequate supply of primary care physicians," says Dr. Chris Ewin, Founder and physician at 121MD in Fort Worth, TX. "This may be true in the country with the correct practice model. Most important, a physician needs to have social skills to sell him/herself and their new practice model to their Patients and their community."

The Top 10 Best States To Start A Career In Concierge Medicine and/or DPC In 2014

Source: The Concierge Medicine Research Collective

1. Utah

2. California

3. Texas

4. Florida

5. Washington State

6. New York

7. Colorado

8. Georgia

9. Tennessee

10. North Carolina

These states were carefully selected based upon internal data and careful analysis where Concierge Medicine and DPC practices are growing. The ability to scale their business for mass-market, employer appeal is likely to occur.

"The reason for the growth of direct access in NY is likely due to the mounting frustration on both the part of the Patients and providers," says Raymond Zakhari, NP and CEO of Metro Medical Direct. "I remember when I started my direct-access, home-based primary care practice (www.MetroMedicalDirect.com) in 2009. Patients were skeptical and reluctant because of how accessible and convenient the service was. They expected to be kept waiting on hold. Some seemed puzzled by the fact that when they called I answered the phone and knew who they were. One Patient even inquired as to how come they only had one form to fill out. Direct-access primary care Patients who have been referred post hospital discharge, have not been readmitted to the hospital in the last 4 years because I can see them without delay or red tape. In NYC, despite the high number of physicians per Patient, particularly on the upper east side of Manhattan, direct-access primary care can still be a viable practice solution for Patients and providers. It helps Patients cut through the red tape that has become expected in accessing health care."

The Top 25 Best Cities To Start A Career in Concierge Medicine and/or DPC in 2014 include:

Source: The Concierge Medicine Research Collective

1. Salt Lake City, UT
2. Provo, UT
3. Los Angeles, CA
4. San Francisco, CA
5. Dallas/Fort Worth, TX
6. San Antonio, TX
7. Miami, FL
8. Fort Lauderdale, FL
9. Seattle, WA
10. New York, NY
11. Denver, CO
12. Colorado Springs, CO
13. Atlanta, GA
14. Nashville, TN
15. Charlotte, NC
16. Chicago, IL
17. Montgomery, AL
18. Birmingham, AL
19. Lincoln, NE
20. Omaha, NE
21. Minneapolis, MN
22. Columbus, OH
23. Boise, ID
24. Nashua, NH
25. Philadelphia, PA

"I think northern GA is a great place to start a DPC (non-third-party) medical practice," said Dr. Robert Nelson who operates a DPC medical practice in Cumming, GA. "Based on conversations I have had with several people in this area since I started my DPC House Call practice, they are definitely open to the idea of innovative changes in healthcare. They are paying attention to trends. It is a diverse economy with an abundance of innovators and business professionals that are looking for an edge to help them personally and professionally. The slow steady economic growth in the region, combined with a diverse population, makes the Forsyth County area of GA a good match for entrepreneurs & innovators in medical care services."

According to a national survey of over 13,000 physicians conducted by Merritt Hawkins on behalf of The Physicians Foundation, 6.8% of physicians in the United States will embrace Concierge Medicine and DPC in the next three years. Business leaders, Concierge Medicine and DPC industry experts and physicians expect the number to be higher – around 15%, according to a recent report by *Concierge Medicine Today*.

"Your overnight success may not last forever, so surround yourself with the right people, possibly the right consultant(s), accountant, attorney and advisers to help you."
-Michael Tetreault, Editor, Concierge Medicine Today

"Being a good physician is not just about knowing how to diagnose and treat disease. Honestly...that's what books and studying is for. Being a good doctor entails earning the trust of your patients by being honest and forthcoming. It means knowing how to communicate effectively while still remaining sympathetic. It requires you, first and foremost, to be a human being. It honestly bothers me that young doctors feel like they have to "know everything" to be a great physician. Put down the damn book and go talk to your patient.
Be a human being. Be a friend. It's really that simple."
- Tiffany Sizemore-Ruiz, D.O. of Choice Physicians of South Florida.

Chapter 2 –
Getting Started.

Being A Tortoise Is Fine.

Private decisions have public consequences. Many physicians who have travelled down the road you are exploring will tell you, this is an important decision that requires a great deal of research, understanding, analysis and wise counsel.

Take it slow. Do your research. This is at least a seven year commitment, minimum. So there is nothing wrong with taking it slow and making the best decision for you, your Patients and your family. Being a tortoise is fine.

When you decided to become a doctor, you went to school to learn. This probably happened in your 20's or maybe into your early 30's. You were in a learning phase. Next, you graduated, applied your learning and as your expertise, personal bedside manner evolved, you adapted to your Patient's needs. You chose those tasks and services that you were passionate about and fine-tuned your practice and place in medicine. This phase probably occurred in your 40's or possibly even in your early 50's. And now, you are in your late 50's/early-mid 60's. Colleagues are coming to you asking you for advice. They are taking you to lunch and want to know 'how you did it?'

Wouldn't it be great if we could just skip all of the years of education, learning and school loan debt that accompanied the learning phase in our career? What if we skipped out on all of those years you had to perfect your craft, visit Patients in the hospital or treat someone before they passed away in the privacy of their own home surrounded by friends, family and loved ones.

Very rarely will success find you by accident. We all search for shortcuts. We all secretly hope there is a backdoor to our dream. But there isn't one. When confronted with work or reward, more often than not, we would choose reward. The secret to starting a Concierge Medicine or DPC practice is that there is no secret. It is an unlocked door. You need to open the door and learn, edit and master the steps.

Whether you are close to retirement age and thinking you would like to end your career with a bit more of a lifestyle advantage or you are in your 30's and thinking what is out there for me? Maybe you are in your 40's and 50's and the business of medicine, Medicare reimbursement and insurance headaches have caused you so much frustration and money over the years that you are thinking of an Encore Career. An Encore Career is work in the second half of life that combines continued income, greater personal meaning, and social impact.

There is a lot to learn from those doctors, office managers and other healthcare pioneers who ventured into an uncertain marketplace before you. They have done so standing in your same shoes. They approached each marketing expenditure and navigational direction with caution and optimism. Because we are not big on impulse purchases, it is more than okay to take things slow and steady. After all, didn't the tortoise win that race?

The Self-Test

Before you take the next step to pursue a Concierge Medicine or DPC model, we have put together the following five criteria to self-evaluate you and your practice before you decided to take the next steps.

Years In Practice.

Doctors, consultants and other industry experts within the Concierge Medicine industry suggest that physicians (of any specialty) should have a minimum of 6 years in private medical practice. However, 10 or more years is preferable.

Your Patient Panel & How Many Patients You Typically See Per Day.

Physicians considering a successful move into a Concierge Medicine practice should have a Patient panel of at least 1,800 Patients that They have seen within the last 24 months. It is also recommended that a minimum of 15 Patients per day are seen across a 4-day period as the current number that your practice is routinely seeing prior to making a transition into Concierge Medicine.

Married Or Unmarried?

Many physicians and their spouses work together in the same office. We found in the practices surveyed that changing your business model requires the agreement of both spouses, whether they work together or not. If your spouse is not in agreement with the change, a transition to a concierge medical practice is not recommended.

Socio-Economic Profile Of Your Current Patients.

While over 62% of current concierge medical programs cost less than $135 per month, the socio-economic profile of Patients in successful Concierge Medicine practices are typically comprised of a majority of middle class / affluent individuals and families.

Age Range Of Current Patients.

According to industry consultants, more than 50% of your current Patient-base (last 24 months) should be 40+ in order to start, sustain and grow a successful Concierge Medicine practice in the future.

Can You Answer 'Yes!' To All Of These Questions?

Whether you choose a consultant or opt to go it alone, these are a few of the common questions you should ask yourself before venturing into this marketplace. If you can answer 'Yes!' to all of the following questions, you are ready to take your curiosity about this model to the next level. The questions are as follows:

1. Have I demonstrated over the year's honesty and financial integrity?
2. Do I have good bedside manner?
3. Have I been there for my Patients when they have needed me most?
4. Do I go beyond the call of duty to help my Patients?
5. Do I actually "like" most of my Patients?
6. Do I have staff that can come with me on this journey?
7. Am I reasonably well-known in my local community as being a high-quality doctor?
8. Do I understand that healthcare quality goes beyond treating the basic medical symptoms I see on a daily basis?
9. Would I be willing to visit my Patients in the hospital?

"The top 4 most popular specialties in Concierge Medicine are: primary care; family medicine; cardiology and pediatrics."

~ Concierge Medicine Today, © 2014

"The top 2 most popular practices' in DPC are: primary care and family medicine. Specialty medicine such as pediatrics, dental, etc., have not found viable cash-only business models in this space in mass yet, in DPC ."

~ The Direct Primary Care Journal, © 2014

"It is a long process," said Helen Hadley, Founder and CEO of VantagePoint Healthcare Advisers in Hamden, CT, which has concierge physician clients. "A practice probably takes as long to start as a [traditional] medical practice."

Time To Start A Business?

"Do not apologize to your Patients for the business changes you are making. This new process will help them. Inform them that this is a positive change and will help you maintain more secure Patient-physician communication on a timely basis and offers them a much more affordable payment system with routine and convenient access to their doctor."
~Mike Permenter, Physician Consultant

We have been covering this industry for a long time. We have kept an eye on many of the Concierge Doctors that have opened since 1996 and watched as many have succeeded beyond their wildest dreams. At the same time, we have seen many Concierge Doctors flounder. They have told us operating and starting a concierge practice was not easy but it is very rewarding. They are so glad they did it. It is not an easy road to follow, but if done properly it can be the most rewarding venture into which you will ever, enter.

Here Is A List Of Important Do's And Don'ts New Concierge Medicine and DPC Doctors When Starting Up Your Practice:

1. Interview your consultant(s) carefully.

Announcing that your medical practice is changing its business model and will now be accepting memberships, retainer-fees or going strictly to a cash-only payment system can be both a scary and exciting adventure. Many physicians we have interviewed over the years tell us it is a challenge but one they are SO HAPPY they pursued. Many Patients will follow them and appreciate having the same friendly doctor but with much greater time and access to his or her services.

You might think that having your Concierge Medicine or DPC practice suddenly overwhelmed with interest and discovered locally or even nationally would be every doctor's dream come true. Yet, too often, that overnight success can quickly become a doctor's worst nightmare. From local media criticism to Patients misunderstanding what you are trying to accomplish with your new business model, a DPC or Concierge Medicine practice that lacks the planning, capital, staff and the operational infrastructure to handle such issues can quickly get crushed when news of so-called 'limited access' becomes a popular theme.

Remember, interview your consultant(s). Always interview at least three or four so you can know what is available to you in the marketplace. We also suggest asking them all the questions you think Patients and staff might ask of you. For example, how long does this process take? What about my EMR System ... will/should it change? What if this does not work out? What then? What is your fee? What is your timeline and implementation strategy to help me do this? Do you have a Patient-practice or Patient-physician service contract I can review? Can you provide references of doctors I can speak to that have utilized your practice transition services in the past year?

Your overnight success may not last forever, so surrounding yourself with the right people, I.e. the right consultant(s), accountant, attorney and advisers to help you can set you up to win in the long run.

2. Do not Go Into Debt By Leasing More Office Space.

While it is only natural to want to celebrate your new practice with a new medical office, remember that Concierge Medicine and DPC physicians' offices usually end up reducing the amount of leased office space they actually need. While it might seem like downsizing your office space is a bad thing, leased office space is the most expensive annual expenditure for Concierge Doctors and DPC physicians so keep your office space at current level or preferably, smaller, not bigger.

3. Do Find A Great Accountant and Fight The Battle on Paper First.

Skipping this step before you start your Concierge Medicine or DPC practice could cause you a lot of frustration. According to industry 'practice conversion' consultants, making a to-do list, crunching the numbers and reviewing your current human capital and operational resources prior to announcing any pricing or business structure change is key. It is always easier to fight a battle on paper (or a computer spreadsheet) than to promote first and having to back-track later. No matter how much pressure you are getting from your consultant, staff or even Patients to deliver new services right now, you need to take the time to sit down with your business partners, spouse, accountants, attorney or staff and map out a strategic business and marketing plan complete with goals, costs and an achievable timeline.

A Concierge Medicine or DPC operation will have to estimate how many additional employees (or in many cases, how many less employees) will be needed to service the expected influx of new faces taking orders on a daily basis over the course of the next year. According to countless interviews over the years with physicians, the average Concierge Medicine medical office employs 1.5 to 2.5 employees, not including the doctor. DPC Clinics typically employ 3-5 employees, not including the doctor, according to *The Direct Primary Care Journal*.

4. Do Prepare Your Staff.

Before you go on a hiring binge and prepare for the influx of phone calls, concerned Patient inquiries and unavoidable angry and tears of joy conversations, it is important to figure out how much working human capital you are going to need to meet your practice demands. Your conversion consultant and/or business advisors and business plan should be able to answer and address all of these questions for you and help train your staff to address these questions and more.

Communication is the lifeblood of any business relationship, but it is even more important when your Concierge Medicine or DPC practice is launched. You should explain to your staff the reasons why this new business model is a good idea. Explain why this will be good for the Patents. Tell them your ideas on transitioning. Those that do not wish to be a part to the practices, explain what it will mean to them. It is important to explain to them what is expected of them: 1) Through the transition; 2) After the transition; 3) The new expectations on how service is rendered to Patients. Prepare them on how to address questions, concerns or angry responses from patients. Get their agreement and buy-in! A staff person not committed to the success of the program because they don't see the value or do not agree with the concept can sabotage your success with patient enrollments.

Once you have worked with your team or consultant to formulate the proper communication, the biggest mistake a doctor can make is failing to explain the value, features and benefits of this new business model to his or her Patients. For example, a Patient's immediate response might be one of great acceptance and they will sign-up with you right away. On the other hand, there will be Patients that might feel like you are abandoning them after years of service. They'll say things like, 'You are just doing this for the money.' Then, you will have to tell them, 'It is not really about that at all, I'm afraid. I am doing this because I want to see my Patients more than just a few minutes each visit and this is a business model that provides you with greater access to me and my staff. It will allow us to maintain greater communication with you and help us help you maintain a healthy lifestyle.'

This can be one of the most scary aspects of conversion but it is one that is necessary. Many 'conversion consultants' can help coach you and your staff through various conversational scenarios that might occur. Sometimes, some consultants will even place an outside person to help you and your staff explain the new model features and benefits in your practice for a few weeks.

Do not commit to hiring full-time employees with payroll taxes and benefits until you are confident your medical office model and strategy is here to stay.

5. **If you build it, they WILL NOT Come. So, invest for the future now.**

While it may be tempting to reap the profits from your new medical business model right away, it is important to re-invest some of those profits to help your business grow and get more Patients. According to interviews over the past five years with Concierge Doctors and DPC physicians and their staff, the number one most successful way they attracted new Patients to their practice was by ... 'hiring a marketing agency' to help with the educational component of your practice.

Bonus Tip! Do not get confused over the difference between what a 'conversion consultant' offers and what 'marketing consultant' or ad agency offers. These are two very different types of consultants. A Marketing Consultant (or Marketing Firm) should have marketplace expertise in both writing and designing materials and effective, lead-generating communication for your practice. Marketing agencies or marketing consultants should offer both offline and online advertising strategies to grow your Patient-base and be able to outline a plan that works with your budget.

A 'Conversion Consultant' is there before you make the switch to help you organize internally, prepare emotionally and plan and staff accordingly as you announce your new business model and pricing structure to your existing Patients. The marketing consultant might be your trusted Patient-referral resource and growth advisor several months after the consultants have left your practice and your annual Patient attrition is beginning to increase. Note the difference?

6. **Learn from your mistakes.**

After the excitement of the initial Patient rush has died down, take some time to sit down with your staff to figure out what went right, what went wrong and what you think you could do better. This will help you put a strategy in place for the future.

7. **Do Decide Whether You Want To Be In A Solo Or Group Practice.**

This is your choice and it is an important one. You should know that the more popular alternative across the U.S. for the past decade has been to open a solo Concierge Medicine practice. Both offer advantages.

In the field of Concierge Medicine, physician surveys and online polling data tells us that 88% of currently operating Concierge Medicine doctors are operating in solo practices while only 12% of Concierge Doctors practice in group settings.

Group settings where there are three or more physicians in the practice and one of those doctors opts or decides to implement a Concierge Medicine or DPC membership program are met with the same challenges legally, ethically and operationally as solo practices. Practices who have one or more doctors considering implementation of this additional service program into their practices are usually met with a fair amount more skepticism and criticism than solo practices. The reason being is that when Patients are offered the choice to continue seeing their current doctor or, pay an extra fee for more time with another doctor in the practice, some Patients are going to think this is unfair and choose the more cost-effective alternative or possibly leave the practice.

Group settings do work though. The doctors relationship with his or her Patients, messaging, marketing, Patient education and staff belief in the program can encourage growth into these add-on membership programs inside group practice settings.

"The challenges of medical center Concierge Medicine programs are very different than those experienced by concierge physicians in private practice.
All hospitals/medical centers have special perks and usually enhanced access to specialists for their donors and patrons, often a special number they can call. Most have an informal "private banking" approach where there is no established fee, just an expected level of donation. Despite the proliferation of individual concierge practices and now organized networks, Concierge Medicine programs INSIDE medical centers are quite unusual – there may be only 20-25 in the entire country."

~ John Kirkpatrick, MD of Seattle, WA
tells Concierge Medicine Today in a recent interview
about Medical Center Concierge Programs

Hospital Environments.

Medical centers are no strangers to Concierge Medicine programs, but they have an entirely different set of complexities to consider when implementing in local hospitals and communities for the first time. The physicians who work inside concierge medical center programs are typically primary care and family physicians and some hospitalists. We know that more hospitals are looking at ways in which they support and service their local communities. More physicians are turning to these facilities for employment.

The Lewis and John Dare Center at Virginia Mason Medical Center in Seattle has been a model for concierge medical care and unique primary care programs for a number of years. In August 2013, the Dare Center invited concierge physicians, hospital administrators and medical center executives from across the country to participate in a roundtable discussion. The inaugural event took place in Seattle, WA.

Representatives from The Lewis and John Dare Center at Virginia Mason Medical Center the discussion. John Kirkpatrick, MD, a Dare Center physician, was one of the main speakers and noted that the focus of the meeting was to bring together staff members of medical centers with existing concierge programs to discuss common problems and share successful solutions. At least 15 medical centers attended this meeting. There was a breakout session for program managers in established practices and another for attendees exploring this type of practice, as well as a roundtable discussion with "lessons learned" from other programs currently operating in the marketplace.

Other topics included: alternative models; amenities/perks; preserving academic standards; legal hurdles; marketing tips; compensation issues; expectations/boundaries; recruiting; networking and other topics important to successful medical center operations.

"The challenges of medical center Concierge Medicine programs are very different than those experienced by concierge physicians in private practice," said Dr. Kirkpatrick. "All hospitals/medical centers have special perks and usually enhanced access to specialists for their donors and patrons, often a special number they can call. Most have an informal private banking approach where there is no established fee, just an expected level of donation. Despite the proliferation of individual concierge practices and now organized networks, Concierge Medicine programs INSIDE medical centers are quite unusual. There may be only 20-25 in the entire country."

The top five considerations institutions should consider when exploring incorporation of Concierge Medicine programs inside medical centers are:

1. The CEO MUST be supportive and the overall organization MUST embrace the concept. This cannot be over-stated.
2. The program needs a Champion. This can be the CEO, or a doctor who is going to provide the care, a VP of Marketing/Business Development, a VP of Foundation or

Development Department. Someone must keep the program moving forward. Someone with the clout to promote and do it.

3. The Medical Center should have a well-to-do population base of interested Patients . This program works for Mayo in the Phoenix, AZ area and in Jacksonville, FL but not Rochester, Minnesota.

4. The Medical Center needs two doctors who already provide personalized services to their Patients.

5. Steering committee of stakeholders – Patients, providers, senior administrators, development officers, marketing experts, nursing staff.

Other very important steps include approval of the legal department and development implementation of an internal marketing plan for education of all staff. This should be performed even before external marketing begun.

If you are considering opening, starting or adding a Concierge Medicine or membership medicine program inside a hospital setting, *Concierge Medicine Today* has relationships and resources that you should consider. Email *Concierge Medicine Today* at editor@conciergemedicinetoday.com and include in the Subject Line: 'Hospital Setting Inquiry.'

"Many concierge practices fail because they try to do it themselves. Even after 10+ years in this still rather exclusive space," says Roberta Greenspan of SpecialDocs, "I continue to have great enthusiasm for the successes and ongoing growth of the concierge model. Every day we hear another story from our physicians and their patients about how much this type of practice change has improved their lives."

The $100,000 Decision and How Others Financed Their Transition.

When Concierge Medicine and DPC doctors across the U.S., were asked 'How Did You Finance Your Concierge or DPC Medical Practice?' The majority of them stated that they paid for the start-up costs associated with transitioning their business model with:

- Personal Assets (savings, house, 401 K, etc.).
- Extra income from shifts at an Urgent Care Center or Emergency Room;
- Credit Union loan;
- Revenue earned or saved from the current practice;
- Crowdsourcing (Kickstarter, Indiegogo, etc.)
- Selling of commercial or personal property.

In no responses were credit cards used to finance start-up costs.

Although concierge medical clinics and DPC doctors' offices are popping up across the country, some hopeful owners are still struggling to get financing. This has many "docpreneurs" wondering how to go about getting the cash they need to either start or maintain their medical business. These days, the application to secure a business loan is extensive and rigorous. According to a recent Pepperdine University survey, nearly two-thirds of privately held, small businesses said they were denied by banks when they applied for a loan. So hopeful physicians have to get creative when it comes to raising money.

One of the most common questions physicians ask when exploring transitioning their practices is 'How much does it cost to transition my insurance-based medical practice to this new Concierge Medicine or DPC business model?'

As previously stated, franchise and consulting fees can move from five-figures to six figures easily. We have learned the average cost is between $150,000 – $250,000 over a period of two to five years and in some rare cases, even longer. Some consultants have quoted figures less than $60,000. However, dependent upon your practice, it is demographics: your bedside manner; Patient surveys (very important); complexity of internal operations; a financial feasibility analysis; and other variables, a Concierge Medicine or DPC practice may or may not be the right option for you.

"Perhaps most important from a doctors perspective," says an industry consultant whose specialty is helping doctors enter into DPC, Mike Permenter, "is that a consulting company should typically furnish all of the capital required to start or modify your medical practice and assumes all risk for success of failure. Thus, the high fees."

As with most of the companies operating in the Concierge Medicine marketplace, a doctor will pay an ongoing fee. Fees can be as low as 15% of each Patient's individual membership fee. However, in most cases it is between 29% to 33% for a period of approximately

3 to 5 years. In some rare cases, up to 25% of the per Patient fee for eight years has been sold to doctors in the southwest part of the U.S. These fees usually include continued support and training in advertising; marketing; sales; operational guidance; technology; legal; regulatory; financial and human resources consulting; and other services.

"Business is tough." says Dr. Chris Ewin of 121MD in Fort Worth, TX. "If you are doing something just for the money, you are never going to enjoy it. You will be the hardest boss you have ever had. So, find something you love and pursue it. Follow this advice and you will set yourself up for an enjoyable future in medicine."

Many doctors start up a Concierge Medicine or DPC practice for a multitude of reasons including: spending more time with Patients; a yearning to use their medical expertise more effectively; a more satisfying lifestyle; and personal reasons. Some doctors enter this field of medicine because they are tired of "hamster" healthcare and frustrated with treadmill medicine that has now become their day job.

Fund It Upfront? Pick Your Payment Poison.

Micro Loans

If you are looking for a loan under $50,000, a microloan may be the way to go. The Small Business Administration's Microloan Program provides small, short-term loans through specially designated intermediary lenders, which are usually nonprofit community-based organizations. While the maximum amount is $50,000, the typical loan is for $13,000. The requirements to obtain a microloan are more lenient as far as your credit score goes. These are helpful when little capital is required as many big banks are generally hesitant to approve loans for under $50,000.

Bank Loans

Before you fill out that bank loan application, do some homework. If you are planning to use a bank loan to get your Concierge Medicine or DPC practice started, run a credit check on yourself. Talk to local bankers about the criteria needed to get a loan. It is very helpful if you have an established relationship with a personal banker or someone at the bank who has been handling or is familiar with your business banking. Then, make sure you have a solid business plan that includes details such as: a competitive analysis; the management process; a marketing analysis and financial projections. Be aware that you will be expected to lay out more of your own cash up front. Banks used to settle for anywhere from 10 percent to 20 percent in cash or assets put up by those seeking a loan. Now they are looking for closer to a 50-50 split, the more money that comes out of your pocket the better as far as they are concerned.

Crowd Funding

Instead of heading to their rich uncle, some are looking into the relatively new phenomenon of "crowd funding". This type of financing is where you get small chunks of funding from everyone in a group such as Kickstarter. This route has a lot lower risk for those involved. The up side is you will have a lot of people with interest in your prospective venture and they may be more likely to give you referrals, possibly become Patients and advise you of opportunities down the road.

What Not to Do

The "don'ts" can be just as important as the "dos" when it comes to financing your Concierge Medicine practice or DPC clinic. Here are three pieces of advice on the subject.

First: do not invest all your time in trying to raise money. There have been many good business concepts that go south because the person has committed everything to raising money and put the concept development on hold.

Second: ideas are great but execution is everything. Do not pursue financing if you do not have a working concept and model.

Lastly, be sure to talk to your financial advisor before making any decision on funding your practice transition. There are always "blind spots" and they may help you identify potential pitfalls of your strategy before you get too far into it. Do not get hung up on the interest rate either. If someone is offering you $50,000 at 12 percent and someone else is offering you $30,000 at 8 percent, the loan with the higher interest rate may be the way to go if that is the capital you need. This may prevent you from spending more than you need.

"It is about believability. Would it work for me? Could it work for me? In places where physicians have taken an early leap of faith [and started a concierge medical practice], they have been satisfied. As a result, physicians now have many examples of colleagues experiencing the benefits of Concierge Medicine for themselves and their Patients. We see momentum continuing to build."

-Richard Doughty, CEO of Cypress Concierge Medicine

About Consultancies —
Consultancies Enter "Red" Ocean

Concierge Medicine consulting firms and individuals once only few in number, are now numbering in the high 30's to 40's.

The competitive sea in the Concierge Medicine consulting marketplace is becoming more crowded. Not for every doctor, DPC practices remain a niche segment of the health care system but consultancies are now registering more physicians than ever.

As industry analysts, journalists, consumer advocates and public relations professionals, see a consultant or company starting to do something that is innovative, we take notice and investigate. What sparked our interest was a concept developed years ago by Renée Mauborgne and W. Chan Kim called *Blue Ocean Strategy*. The blue ocean is a metaphor for companies operating in uncontested market space.

In the early 2000's, the Concierge Medicine marketplace was predominantly serviced by two or three consulting companies. In 2010, the number increased to over 20. Today that number has grown into the high 30's to 40's.

Large franchise companies, like MDVIP, continue to capture a significant portion of the market share. They still have an edge, in that they helped build the existing sea in which they now sail. These franchise Concierge Medicine consultancies like MDVIP and Concierge Choice help to keep prices low and competitive for not just their physician clients but their Patient members as well.

In 2007, P&G acquired a 48% stake in MDVIP, a Concierge Medicine company that was formed in 2000. Then, in December 2009, Procter & Gamble acquired 100% ownership in MDVIP for an undisclosed sum. See "Boutique Medicine Venture Generates Marketing Intelligence for Procter & Gamble", February 4, 2010. In April/May of 2014, Proctor and Gamble announced it was selling MDVIP to Summit Partners, a private equity firm. MDVIP is the largest concierge medical company with over 700 practices across the U.S. and more than thousands of Patient subscribers.

Other successful, less franchised consultancies such as Specialdocs, Cypress Concierge Medicine and a select few others continue to innovate, offering differing models, competitive fees and personal service within a doctor's practice.

"Even after 10+ years in this still rather exclusive space," says Roberta Greenspan of Specialdocs, "I continue to have great enthusiasm for the successes and ongoing growth of the concierge model. Every day we hear another story from our physicians and their Patients about how much this type of practice change has improved their lives."

Currently, there is a phenomenal opportunity for these companies to innovate and sail into clearer, bluer waters. We frequently hear from Concierge Medicine and DPC physicians who are frustrated with their consultant or transition experience. There is definitely a way for existing and future consultants to improve on service and price. Dyson made vacuum cleaners a tech-gadget with its futuristic design and disposing with flimsy one-use filters. Concierge Medicine consulting companies can and most likely will, incorporate a service, price or technology-that will be just as unique?

Companies like MedFirst Partners, Specialdocs, Inc., and Cypress Concierge Medicine are already bringing innovation and highly personalized service into this niche space. But when the most common complaints heard about the DPC consulting and franchise Concierge Medicine industry is poor customer service, ongoing management fees, lack of support following the initial transition and high prices, companies servicing the marketspace must begin offering something truly unique to their physician clients as they are now entering the competitive phase of market development.

"The first thing to decide is whether you want to continue billing insurance," says Mike Permenter, long-time industry consultant and physician advisor. "If so, then there are specific legal issues to address with regards to the structure. If you are opting out of insurance there are a number of options. The biggest mistake in my opinion is charging too low. Conversions [into this private-pay marketplace] will eventually be unnecessary as the public becomes more aware of the benefits of these types of memberships. The big challenge is continuing growth after the initial conversion. Customer service, as described by some physicians, is the number one way to grow [this type of] practice. Linking the service to local self-insured employers is a good way to grow but certainly requires expertise with regards to structuring the appropriate benefit, usually a high-deductible plan with an HSA plus a membership. Most doctors currently practicing concierge medicine as a career choice fall into one of two intelligence-gathering categories when they first opened. First, they used a franchise concierge company to help them with the details or they opted to do it themselves and surround themselves with a local team that would provide counsel in starting this practice model. I perform a thorough analysis of the practice and determine areas where expenses will be reduced. After a survey of the physician's patients, we conduct a 12-16 week conversion. Our fees are collected during the transition only. Once a successful conversion has been completed, we help train the physician staff to provide membership services. If customer service is maintained, we know the practice will continue growing without a need for further services." -Mike Permenter, long-time industry consultant and physician advisor.

Nancy Latady of Latady Physician Strategies addresses this and says "for the implementation phase – the actual practice conversion – we either do everything for them (holding their hand throughout the process), or we provide coaching if they want to do most of it themselves. Our primary goal is to help physicians transition their practices successfully – by doing it right the first time, resulting in more Patients, more quickly, and to achieve greater profitability."

We know that physicians are being offered intolerable reimbursements from traditional insurance and health plan relationships. Years ago, 120% of the Medicare fee schedule was considered to be a frightfully low reimbursement. Insurers and managed care networks are now offering reimbursements at 75% of Medicare Rates or even lower in some extreme cases.

The language of strategy rather than the delivery of platitudes are more informative and effective with physicians when talking to them about how Concierge Medicine will benefit their practice, Patients and bottom-line. For consultants to sail and compete in the Concierge Medicine ocean over the next two to four years, the company that will repeatedly give its physician clients something that feels refreshingly new and solves their problems in a way no existing consultant has done will exit the red ocean and begin trawling in blue waters.

Cypress Concierge Medicine is a Louisiana based healthcare consulting company that specializes in Concierge Medicine transitions. Cypress is unique in that it does not own or directly manage physician practices. Instead, they provide direction, oversight, regulatory support and control, ongoing legal review and the expertise necessary for a physician to provide a positive experience for each Patient encounter.

"With Concierge Medicine, the impact for Patients and physicians is phenomenal," says Richard Doughty, CEO in a recent article on Baton Rouge's *The Advocate*.

"One of the reasons behind the company's success is that it offers doctors the personal touch," Doughty said. *"That approach gives doctors confidence in the company. Cypress does not want to lose its person-to-person quality or make physicians feel like each one isn't important."*

Doughty attributes all of his success, past and future, to his faith. Cypress' growth is really up to God, adds the article. "I will tell you this ... God is doing some amazing things," Doughty said. "I just do not want to limit Him."

The paper adds, the *company offers two key advantages over competitors: a lower-cost fee structure and the ability to tailor a practice model to the physician and his or her Patients.*

"In a typical concierge practice, the management firm gets one-third of the membership fees Patients pay," Doughty said. *"Most contracts are for five years, and the fee structure remains the same over the life of the contract. If a practice has 600 members and the members pay $1,500 a year, the management firm's share is $300,000 a year. Over a five-year contract, that adds up to $1.5 million. But most of the heavy lifting is done*

during the first 18 months of moving the practice to the concierge model. After that, if the management firm has done a good job, there is not nearly as much work required. Cypress drops its fees each year, in proportion to the amount of effort and energy required to maintain the practice. The difference for doctors generally amounts to several hundred thousand dollars over the course of a contract."

Cypress Concierge Medicine offers three practice models, Doughty adds.

- A straight concierge practice.
- A blended model under which the physician maintains his practice's current Patient population, but personally sees only the Patients that join the concierge practice. The doctor oversees nurse practitioners or physicians assistants, who manage the non-concierge Patients.
- A block-time model, where the physician dedicates a certain portion of the day to concierge Patients and the rest to traditional Patients.

The number of physicians signing on with concierge practice companies continues to increase. A report by Merritt Hawkins, a physician staffing firm, found that nearly 10 percent of practice owners planned to convert to concierge practices over the next three years. The Concierge Medicine Research Collective ("The Collective") estimates Concierge Medicine and DPC physician's number to be approximately 12,000 in the U.S. and Canada. This is according to analyses and a recent examination of the national marketplace by The Collective as well as interviews with corporate industry leaders.

"I knew I was being compromised by seeing Patients every eight to ten minutes just to keep the doors open."

-Dr. Jack Padour, Ventura, CA.

Three Year Analysis Of Concierge And Direct Care Medicine Shows Encouraging Signs For Boosting Primary Care In U.S. Economy

© 2013, *The Concierge Medicine Research Collective*, ConciergeMedicineToday.com

In 2013, *Concierge Medicine Today* released a 3-year (2009-2012) summary of its analysis on the popularity and growth of the Concierge Medicine and DPC marketplace. They asked physicians throughout the U.S. from December 2009 to December 2012 questions pertaining to their Concierge Medicine and DPC practice, Patient satisfaction, business strategies, revenues and more. The analysis revealed the following results:

- Nearly 70% of current U.S. Concierge Medicine and DPC physicians operating practices today are internal medicine specialists.
- The second most popular medical specialty in Concierge Medicine is family practice.
- A surprising finding in this study was the increasing number of concierge cardiology, dental and pediatric practices opening from February of 2010 to December 2012.
- The combined average annual income of a typical Concierge Medicine [and direct care] Patient is between $50,000 to $200,000 per year.
- Average annual compensation/salary of Concierge Doctor is between $100,000 and $300,000 per year.
- The typical age of Concierge Doctor is between 40-59 years of age.
- 77% of a concierge [and DPC] Patients are between the age of 40-59 years old.
- A Concierge Medicine doctor who provides 24/7 cell phone access receives the majority (83%) of phone calls from their Patients during normal business hours, Monday through Friday.
- 62% of direct care and concierge medical offices employ between 1-2 office employees.
- The most common reason why Concierge Medicine Patients call their doctors: Prescription Renewals (38%); Cold/Flu Symptoms (19%); Back Pain (14%); and Headaches (13%).
- Most Concierge Doctors and DPC physicians treat six to eight Patients per day.
- More than 70% of concierge [and DPC] doctors will visit with their Patients between 30-60 minutes per office visit, enough time to discuss case history, examination, other symptoms, treatment options and strategy for care.
- Patients using Concierge Medicine [and DPC] comply with scripts and recommendations far more due to the doctor's routine personal follow-up with the Patients and explaining the importance of compliance and other treatment options.

The analysis looked at Concierge Medicine's growth, the business models used, popular trends, and a wide variety of physician surveys, interviews and secure polling data on a number of aspects pertaining to the average Concierge Medicine and DPC practice. Doctors who practice internal medicine and family medicine are by choice and nature, treating nearly 90% of a Patients' healthcare concerns, ailments and illnesses each year. For over a decade, Concierge Medicine has had a love-hate relationship with the public. The public loves the idea or loathes it, but a lot of people are coming around. However, if they truly understand it, there is nothing that quite compares to it. It is an educational curve we are overcoming in the marketplace on a national level with analysis and education like this.

Many doctors fly under the radar. *Concierge Medicine Today* believes the growth rate will be high in the coming years – possibly as high as 15%+ of primary care doctors due to the Affordable Care Act (ACA). In 2013 alone, industry sources and concierge consultants tell us that they have seen as significant increase in physician interest to support this growth.

According to The Collective, Concierge Medicine doctors and DPC clinics across the U.S. now serve over 240,600 Patients (June 2013).

As more and more companies and individuals sail in these waters and seek to find their catch, inevitably this will mean price competition and ultimately, the physicians moving into these practices will benefit the most.

Fight The Battle on Paper First.

Skipping this step before you start your Concierge Medicine or DPC practice could cause you a lot of frustration. According to industry 'practice conversion' consultants, making a to-do list, crunching the numbers and reviewing your current human capital and operational resources prior to announcing any pricing or business structure change is key. It is always easier to fight a battle on paper (or a computer spreadsheet) than to promote first and ask questions later. No matter how much pressure you are getting from your consultant, staff or even Patients to deliver new services right now, you need to take the time to sit down with your business partners, spouse, accountants, attorney or staff to map out a strategic business and marketing plan complete with goals, costs and an achievable timeline.

A concierge-style or direct-pay operation will have to estimate how many additional employees (or, in many cases, how many less employees) will be needed to service the expected influx of new faces taking orders on a daily basis over the course of the next year. According to *Concierge Medicine Today*'s interviews over the years, the average Concierge Medicine medical office employs 1.5 to 2.5 employees (2010-2012).

Buy The Building? Do not Go Into Debt By Leasing More Office Space.

"Looking back I would have purchased the building we are in instead of renting." says Atlanta area concierge physician, Dr. Edward Espinosa of Buckhead Concierge Internal Medicine.

Conversely, it is only natural to want to celebrate your new practice with a new medical office. Remember that Concierge Medicine and DPC physicians usually end up reducing the amount of leased office space they actually need. While it might seem like downsizing your office space is a bad thing, leased office space is the most expensive annual expenditure for Concierge Doctors and DPC physicians followed by staff payroll.

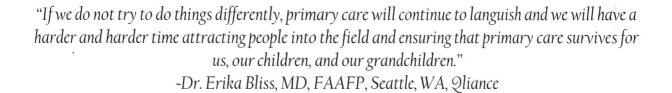

"If we do not try to do things differently, primary care will continue to languish and we will have a harder and harder time attracting people into the field and ensuring that primary care survives for us, our children, and our grandchildren."
~Dr. Erika Bliss, MD, FAAFP, Seattle, WA, Qliance

Our analysis also found that there are currently four states that have a huge lead in the amount of active concierge physicians in practice and consumers seeking their services. Florida, California, Pennsylvania and Virginia each have a significant number of people seeking out concierge and DPC doctors and there is, fortunately, a sizeable number of concierge physicians to serve them. Most of these Patients are over age 50.

While the number of physicians entering concierge medical practices needs to increase, expanded geographic coverage availability is needed. Through *DOC FINDER*, we are learning that the number of Patients who are seeking concierge medical care is far greater than the actual number of primary care and family practice doctors available to serve them. This data, as well as other studies, tells us that it is extremely difficult to find a concierge or DPC doctor in rural areas such as: Idaho; North and South Dakota; Louisiana; Mississippi; New Hampshire and others. Oftentimes, we are learning that there are less than a half dozen practitioners to serve an entire state.

Our analysis also discovered that three out of every eight Concierge Doctors that are incorporating unique anti-aging and medical home solutions into their practices from 2012 to 2013 are seeing their Patients nearly two to three times more each year than a traditional Concierge Medicine and DPC practice.

Since the election in November 2012, *DOC FINDER* has also seen a tremendous increase in the amount of interest, inquiries and physician searches across the U.S. People are concerned about the Affordable Care Act, access to their physician and unsure about future costs. Doctors are adapting. They are hearing from their Patients about what is successful and learning exactly what is appealing to their audience and local Patients. Most doctors are communicating daily, weekly and monthly -- with the majority of Patients in a Concierge Medicine and DPC clinic and that strategy is proving to be beneficial year after year.

Financially, the three year analysis asked doctors 'How is your practice performing financially with Concierge Medicine and DPC Patients?' Surprisingly, these physicians show improvement each since 2008 year, despite the country's slow economic recovery.

- Seventy-one percent (71%) of all current Concierge Medicine and DPC physicians are doing 'Better' financially than 2008;
- Twenty-four percent (24%) indicated 'No Change' and;
- Thirteen percent (13%) indicated they were doing 'Worse.'

"More time with Patients practicing prevention IS better care. I dare any doc to deny that ..."

-Dr. Sarah M. Gamble, D.O., a Concierge Doctor in Greenwich, CT

Chapter 3
Planning And Preparation.

We have had the pleasure of developing relationships with countless physicians, industry consultants and the media over the past several years. We have interviewed just about every industry analyst, interviewed countless physicians and industry consultants and heard just about every opinion you could imagine on the topic of Concierge Medicine and DPC. We keep in touch with hundreds of doctors that have successful practices and we have equipped, educated, counseled, coached, and observed as many of them have succeeded beyond their wildest dreams.

At the same time, we have seen many Concierge Doctors flounder. Regardless of who you talk to in the marketplace, doctor, consultant or staff. They will all tell you one thing ... 'running a concierge practice is not an easy road to follow, but if done properly it can be the most rewarding venture you will ever enter into.'

A Few Business Tips For The First Time Private-Pay, Direct Care And Concierge Medicine Doctor

1.   **Communicate With Your Patients Often And Early.**

Communication is the lifeblood of any business relationship, but it is even more important when your Concierge Medicine practice is being launched. Once you have worked with your trusted team of advisors or conversion consultant to formulate the proper strategy, letters, printed promotional materials, met with your staff, educated them on how to present your new practice model, and you have approved your strategic plan, the biggest mistake a doctor can make now is failing to communicate with his or her Patients. They must be informed early that your business model is changing and that there is a deadline in which to join. Beyond the deadline, it might be too late. Remember, the majority of Concierge Medicine and retainer-based practices limit their Patient-base to approximately 300-600 Patients each year.

2.   **Do Not Apologize To Your Patients For The Business Changes You Are Making.**

This new business model and process will help them. Inform them that this is a very positive change that will help you maintain more frequent Patient-Physician contact, initiate communications on a timely basis and offers a more affordable payment system with routine and convenient access to their doctor. This will allow you to have the time to help them stay well and healthy for the future.

This can be one of the scariest aspects of conversion but it is one that is necessary. Some consultants can help coach you and your staff through various conversational scenarios that might occur. Sometimes, some consultants will even place an outside person in your practice to help you and your staff explain the new model features and benefits in your practice for a time.

A Patient's immediate response to this concept might be one of great acceptance and they will sign-up with your right away. On the other hand, there will be Patients that may object to your new model feel like you are abandoning them after years of service. They will say things like, 'You are just doing this for the money.' Then, you will have to tell them, 'It is not really about that at all. I am doing this because I want to see my Patients more than just a few minutes each visit. This is a business model that offers greater access to me and my staff, and it allows us to maintain greater communication with you and work more closely with you to stay healthy for the years to come.'

3.   Stop Hiring Like A Start-Up Concierge Practice

Over the past several years, we have spent countless hours in interviews, conducting surveys and learning from all types of physicians and practice models what it takes to survive, thrive and grow a successful Concierge Medicine and DPC practice. But there is always one concern that is been a popular topic over the years in this environment and that is ... staffing and turnover inside Concierge Medicine or DPC doctors' offices.

As a young start-up Concierge Medicine or DPC clinic, you probably discontinued several of your insurance and managed care relationships and, consequently, reduced the amount of staff you need to operate. When it is time to hire someone to replace or add to your concierge medical or DPC health team, it is not uncommon to spend several hours a day over a long period of time reviewing resumes, doing background checks and scheduling telephone and in-person interviews.

In addition to the sheer volume of resumes you will receive, the growing pains associated with transitioning from a small startup concierge practice to a medium-sized, thriving and successful company are many. Most Concierge Medicine practices only employ 1-3 people, according to *The Concierge Medicine Research Collective*.

The Fix: Rather than micro-managing the hiring process, concierge physicians should shift some staffing responsibilities to their managers. When your practice has moved past the one-man-band that helped launch you to where you are today, physicians should seek out specialists to help meet their hiring goals. In today's Concierge Medicine and direct care practice, managers carry lot of responsibility and are, in most cases, the best way to ensure that your practice hires the right person with the right skillsets. Many can be evaluated through tests like those given to computer developers to gauge their problem-solving skills and overall knowledge. This action can help vet your hiring candidates before you, the physician or owner of the practice, ever need to be involved. Interviews for new hires nowadays can occur via Skype as well.

As your practice grows, your human resources can become more formalized. According to Entrepreneur.com, check-ins with new staff should happen at multiple intervals, after the first and second weeks as well as after the first 30, 60 and 90 days to ensure they have the tools they need and can get questions answered.

Now, with the use of your manager dedicated to helping you in the new hire process, you should spend less than two hours a week on talent acquisition and hiring.

"I want an entrepreneurial culture," says one concierge physician from New York City. "Hiring is part of growing and we need to make sure our type of practice Concierge Medicine does it right. We have a lot to live up to as Concierge Doctors. Let's get our employees' attitude and service capabilities right."

Takeaway Point

A large, rapidly growing concierge medical practice or DPC practice must evolve its hiring practices and empower staff to take the reins.

"We probably turn away 60%-70% of the doctors who approach us," says Roberta Greenspan, Founder of Specialdocs Consultants, based in Chicago, IL "It is not how much money the Patient has in their bank account; it is how loyal they are, how strong their feelings are for the physician," she explains. "Patients will say, 'I didn't really want to pay $1800 a year for a membership fee. That is a lot of extra money when I'm already paying so much for health insurance. But I'll do it because I do not want to leave Dr. Smith. He means the world to me.'"

Top 10 Fastest Growing Cities For Concierge Medicine

© 2013-2014, *The Concierge Medicine Research Collective*, ConciergeMedicineToday.com

1. Los Angeles, CA
2. San Francisco, CA
3. New York, NY
4. Palm Beach, FL
5. Baltimore, MD
6. Washington, DC
7. Philadelphia, PA
8. Seattle, WA
9. Chicago, IL
10. San Diego, CA

- The combined average annual income of a typical Concierge Medicine [and direct care] Patient is between $50,000 to $200,000 per year.
- Most Concierge Doctors and DPC physicians treat six to eight Patients per day.
- More than 60% of Concierge Medicine and DPC subscriptions/membership fees cost less than $135 per month.

"If you are going to do a comprehensive wellness exam on everyone once a year, it takes an hour or two," says Dr. Thomas LaGrelius, a direct pay physician in California. "You can only do about three a day and take care of everyone else's medical problems. That limits you to a membership base of about 600 Patients — maybe 800 if they are younger, healthier people."

In a recent *MedScape* article written by Neil Chesanow, he cites that Specialdocs Consultants, Inc., (Specialdocs), a health care consulting firm dedicated to transitioning traditional medical practices to personalized, custom-designed concierge medicine models....and providing ongoing support for those practices already transitioned, has 2 important questions for prospective physicians: "How long have you been in the community where you are currently practicing? How many Patients have you seen in the past two years?" Greenspan says. "These are so important because the loyalty factor trumps everything."

The article continues to add ... As an indicator of Patient loyalty, Specialdocs considers whether prospective clients have been in practice in the same community for a minimum of 8 years, but preferably 10 years or longer. If the doctor is a primary care physician, a panel of about 1600 Patients over a 2-year period is also desirable. That is because, even with long-time Patients, only a fraction will opt to pay an annual fee — which, among Specialdocs clients, averages about $1800 per year. Established in 2002, Specialdocs has successfully transitioned more than 150 medical practices nationwide, including internal medicine practices and specialties such as cardiology, endocrinology, pulmonology, pediatrics and women's health.

Chesanow also points out that a consultant establishes the legal basis for offering non-covered services by a concierge practice, recruits Patients, trains doctor and staff in how to deliver Patient-friendly service, if necessary, and handles billing and collections for the annual membership fees that Patients pay to belong. Concierge consultants do not generally get involved in the clinical side of a client practice.

In addition, concierge practices commonly offer lectures, workshops, and clinics as part of the annual fee. Depending on doctor and Patient interests, these may include diet, nutrition, yoga, and cosmetics classes; acupuncture; ultrasonography; physical therapy; sports medicine testing; group counseling for Patients with chronic disease; and wellness seminars.

The *MedScape* article states:

Before deciding to transition, [Dr. Thomas] LaGrelius had his expert perform a demographic analysis of his conventional panel to see whether there was likely to be enough Patients to support a full concierge practice. Surveys were conducted to gauge the level of Patient interest. Patients received announcement letters, brochures, and other promotional materials created by the marketing firm. The firm also trained LaGrelius and his staff in the niceties of concierge service, stationed a representative in the old practice to explain the benefits of the new practice to Patients after their visits with the doctor, and installed a direct phone line to the firm's headquarters in Chicago, enabling Patients to call Specialdocs for answers to their questions while they were still in the office.

"Every Patient whom I talked to, I would get on the phone or refer them to that line and the consultant would describe to them what the practice was going to be like and sell it to them,"

LaGrelius says. "She actually explained it and sold it and was incredibly effective at that. It was very labor-intensive." Source: Concierge Practices Even for Doctors Who Do not Like the Idea. *Medscape*. Jan 09, 2014. http://www.medscape.com/viewarticle/818644

Legal Issues

NOTE: This section does not constitute as legal advice. Individuals, businesses, physicians and others needing and seeking professional advice and counsel should consult their attorney.

With the advice and counsel of a trusted attorney who understands healthcare law in your state, avoiding and overcoming the legal challenges presented by starting a DPC or Concierge Medicine practice is achievable.

Michael L. Blau, head of the Health Law Department at McDermott, Will & Emery in Boston, MA, was quoted in a story published by *Medical Economics* as saying that the key to avoiding the ban on balance billing and other pitfalls brought on by starting a Concierge Medicine or DPC practice is to draw a very bright line between the non-covered Concierge Medicine and/DPC services for which you are collecting a fee, and the covered services for which you are billing payers and/or Medicare.

The article in *Medical Economics* also noted ... *Concierge Medicine and DPC practices that continue to bill insurers should consider setting up "a wholly separate business entity [corporation] alongside their professional corporation. The business corporation, which is "not authorized to engage in the practice of medicine," collects the non-covered fees; the professional corporation, which is authorized to practice medicine, "accepts payment in full for covered services from third-party payers, subject to co-insurance, deductibles, and copays."*

A complex financial relationship between the two entities" permits the revenue from one to be shared by the other. Doctors who go the franchise route circumvent this legal thicket, since the franchise company itself services as the separate business corporation.

Doctors must also be careful when discontinuing and terminating relationships with current Patients, particularly those with a "continuing, intensive course of treatment," notes Blau. He advises meeting with Patients to discuss their options prior to sending out any form of communication or letter announcing your move into Concierge Medicine, retainer-based medicine or DPC healthcare. "If doctors do this, there shouldn't be any continuity of care or Patient abandonment issues," he says.

Concierge Medicine Raises Legal Issues

Attorney, Michael H. Cohen of the Michael H. Cohen Law Group says ...

Concierge or boutique medical practices raise legal issues requiring knowledge of insurance laws, contract legal issues, and ethical rules applicable to medical doctors and other clinicians.

Concierge Medicine, retainer medicine, involves charging Patients or clients subscription (or access) fees for medical and other health care services.

Frequently physician entrepreneurs will create a model of high-end, primary care through Concierge Medicine, but be unaware of the legal pitfalls from laws relating to insurance, contracts, and so on.

One of the key legal issues is the extent to which the access or retainer fee for the concierge medical practice includes services that are routinely covered by insurance — such as physical exams, routine medical office visits, and routine diagnostic tests.

Typically, the practice is on safer legal ground when it includes only medical services that are typically not covered by insurance.

The insurance legal problem is most thorny where Medicare is involved. If the concierge practice charges Patients an access fee for services that are covered under Medicare, federal enforcement authorities could see this as violating Medicare rules. In such case, the safest legal strategy may be to simply opt-out of Medicare. Opting out of Medicare, however, requires precisely following the opt-out rules set by Medicare. It is not a default; the default mode is to be non-participating (or non-par), which still subjects the medical doctor to Medicare rules. Physicians often get caught in the regulatory cross-hairs by failing to properly fill out the proper forms, failing to properly inform their Patients, billing when they are not supposed to, communicating poorly with their Medicare carrier, or thinking they are opted out when they are simply non-par. Medicare billing violations are common and the legal consequences are steep. The Office of the Inspector General (OIG) has warned that substantial penalties and exclusions from federal health care reimbursement programs may apply. The risk is even greater for a participating physician.

Services that are non-covered by Medicare do not raise the same red legal red flag for a concierge medical practice. However, it is sometimes difficult to determine whether the proposed medical service is a covered or non-covered one under Medicare, as there are large areas of overlap. Where Medicare specifically exempts a given service, this creates a clearer legal situation. It is important to note that physicians can be reimbursed for non-covered services if the Medicare Patient signs an Advance Beneficiary Notice (ABN), acknowledging that some services may not be covered by Medicare and that if Medicare denies coverage, the beneficiary must pay the physician for the medical service.

Of course, if the doctor is not under Medicare then the issue arises not under Medicare but under the private insurance agreements where the clinician is under contract. These must be carefully analyzed by an attorney familiar with insurance law who can help navigate through the various contractual provisions at stake.

A second issue that arises is that of illegal kickbacks and fee-splitting legal rules. When concierge practices offer "free" services this raises concerns under the federal anti-kickback statute (AKS) if Medicare is involved, and otherwise and additionally under state anti-kickback laws. The "free" service can be viewed by enforcement authorities as an illegal inducement for clinical services. There is usually a "fair market value" safe harbor which can be utilized; however, the transaction must be carefully scrutinized for legal compliance.

The third issue is whether the access fee could be considered the practice of insurance, and therefore subject the entity or medical practice offering the pre-paid medical service to state regulation as an insurer. It is possible that fee-for-service arrangements will be viewed as outside insurance regulations; however, access fees for prepaid services can raise legal issues.

Sometimes it is helpful to contact the state insurance commissioner and/or managed care departments. Some states have exceptions for prepayment or "fast payment" arrangements.

Whether or not the concierge, boutique, or direct access practice is deemed the business of insurance under state law, there could be other state insurance regulations that apply to the practice. For example, there could be concerns about balance billing. Once again, non-covered services may pose less of a legal issue for insurance commissioners at the state level; and fee-for-service may be less risky than providing unlimited access or prepaid clinical services for a flat fee.

Fourth, the arrangement must comply with any contractual arrangements the entity or provider has with private insurance companies or third-party payers, as noted. For example, the private insurance company may have a clause that prohibits balance billing – i.e., billing the Patient for a service after or in lieu of the rate of reimbursement allowed by the insurance agreement. The prohibition on balance billing usually only applies to covered services so there may be an "out" here. Once again, the contract should be carefully reviewed by an attorney familiar with insurance contracts in the medical arena. Deciding to not accept insurance is one option, although that may reduce overall revenues.

Another concern is how to terminate Patients after a set level of services has been provided. State laws and ethical rules prohibit Patient abandonment. The Patient must be given enough time to find a new and satisfactory physician.

Concierge medical practices must also be aware of advertising laws applicable to physicians and non-physician providers (both allied health and complementary and alternative medicine practitioners), and also refrain from claims of effectiveness, result, and cure that cannot be realized and may only accelerate potential liability. An experienced attorney can review marketing materials for compliance with relevant laws and to help minimize potential liability exposure.

In general, the concierge practice would benefit not only from clear legal review by an experienced health care and contracts attorney, but also by having the lawyer draft a contract between the practice and the Patient that clearly specifies the services to be covered by the access or subscription fee; the Medicare status of the physicians involved; whether those providers accept insurance; how the billing will be done; and what will happen when the Patient is terminated from the program.

Another concern that arises is when non-physician practices try to package clinical services (such as, for example, acupuncture) and non-clinical, spa services. For example, the wellness center offers the client a package. The package consists of 10 sessions: 3 acupuncture sessions, 2 massage therapy sessions, and 5 sessions in the infrared sauna. The client will prepay for all 10 sessions. The question is whether this practice violates some of the above legal rules.

There are several issues here. One is whether the above rules relevant to concierge medical practices will similarly apply to non-physician practices such as acupuncture (or chiropractic, massage, naturopathic medicine, psychology, counseling, and hypnotherapy and other services). The answer depends in part on state law and what arrangements the clinician has with insurance.

Another area of legal inquiry is whether conflating clinical and non-clinical services raises kickback or fee-splitting issues, or subjects the clinician to potential charges of exceeding scope of practice. For example, suppose the only arrangement is one in which the Patient pre-purchases acupuncture visits, but can see any acupuncturist in the practice. The question is whether this involves fee-splitting or a kickback, in that the discount could potentially be viewed as an illegal inducement (or incentive) from acupuncturist A to see acupuncturist B (especially if A owns the clinic).

CPM, the corporate practice of medicine, may also be triggered if state law applies this legal rule to professions outside of medicine and views the arrangement as the entity itself interfering with clinical practice.

Yet another potential area of law is that applicable to gift cards, since state law could have legal rules regarding discounts and packaged services.

Once again, the arrangement must be structured carefully by an attorney well-versed in corporate practice of medicine, fee-splitting and kickback laws, insurance law, and other legal rules, so that the transaction passes legal muster and is legally compliant.

"If you can opt-out of Medicare, financially, emotionally and otherwise, Concierge Medicine might be a good option to pursue," he explains.
"But for the doctor who says he does not want to leave his Medicare Patients, that is a big fork in the road – and a major consideration."

- Jack Marquis, Attorney, Warner, Norcross & Judd

Four Questions to Ask Before You Transition

Attorney Jack Marquis of Warner, Norcross & Judd in a 2012 *Concierge Medicine Today* article writes ... The concierge model of medicine has grown significantly over the last decade, but a Warner Norcross & Judd LLP attorney encourages physicians to ask four key questions before making the transition. Health lawyer, Jack Marquis said that the concierge model continues to attract physicians who want to provide more focused care to a smaller number of Patients than typically served in a traditional medical practice. Also known as retainer-based medicine, boutique practices [DPC], and innovative medical practice design, concierge practices vary widely in structure, but typically offer Patients enhanced access to their physician via 24/7 phone calls, same-day or next-day appointments, e-mail communications, and other benefits in exchange for a monthly or annual retainer [fee].

"Concierge Medicine continues to be a growth industry," said Marquis, who has helped scores of physicians and physician practices make the transition. "There are benefits to Patients and physicians alike, but I caution doctors who are contemplating the switch to examine their practices before making a leap. Answering a few questions will be key in determining if a concierge model is right for your specific practice."

Marquis also notes that physicians need to consider the following four important questions before converting their practice into a concierge medical office. Those include:

Where do you live? Physicians need to be sure they live in a community with a large enough population base to support the transition from a traditional to a concierge practice.

Can you opt out of Medicare? While there are many varieties of concierge practices, Marquis notes that they come down to two basic types: Those that accept Medicare and those that do not. "If you can opt out of Medicare, financially, emotionally and otherwise, Concierge Medicine might be a good option to pursue," he explains. "But for the doctor who says he does not want to leave his Medicare Patients, that is a big fork in the road – and a major consideration."

Do you have enough Patients? Physicians need to determine if they have enough Patients willing to transition with them to create a sustainable business model. "This is the biggest angst that doctors go through before making a transition," Marquis noted. "It becomes a matter of how risky is it for you when you do not really know?"

Are you willing to be aggressive with marketing? Marquis noted that the single biggest key to successful transitions he has seen over the last decade is having an ongoing marketing program – not just advertising. "It is critical to keep new Patients coming into the practice. That means physicians need to utilize all marketing tools available to them, such as existing Patients, web sites, the media, etc."

"The new Act presents a much more fundamental problem for FNCS practices by creating a new Medicare-covered service called Personalized Preventive Plan Services, now being called by CMS simply the Annual Wellness Visit (the "AWV")."

- Jack Marquis, Attorney, Warner, Norcross & Judd

Recommended Reading

New Health Care Act Removes Legal Justification For Most FNCS Concierge Practices
By Jack R. Marquis | WNJ | Legal | 04-1-2011

Jack Marquis has more than forty years' experience in business, tax and health law.
He founded the firm's Concierge Medicine practice and has helped physicians across the country
establish these practices. Recently he was named 2013 Tax Lawyer of the Year in the
Grand Rapids, MI area by the Best Lawyers in America publication.

Available at: www.ConciergeMedicineToday.com

"Typically, the concierge medical practice is on safer legal ground when it includes only medical services that are typically non-covered by insurance."
- Michael H. Cohen, Attorney

Recommended Reading

Concierge Medicine V. DPC: Legal Issues
By Michael H. Cohen, Attorney, Michael H. Cohen Law Group, www.michaelhcohen.com

Michael H. Cohen is a thought leader in health care law, pioneering legal strategies and solutions for clients in traditional and emerging healthcare markets. Read more at:
http://michaelhcohen.com

Available at: www.ConciergeMedicineToday.com

"Both Concierge Medicine and DPC can implicate Stark, federal anti-kickback law, and federal and state self-referral, anti-kickback, and fee-splitting laws."
- Michael H. Cohen, Attorney

Recommended Reading

How Medicare.Gov Helps With Legal Review of Concierge Medicine Services
By Michael H. Cohen, Attorney, Michael H. Cohen Law Group, www.michaelhcohen.com

Michael H. Cohen is a thought leader in health care law, pioneering legal strategies and solutions for clients in traditional and emerging healthcare markets. Read more at: http://michaelhcohen.com

Available at: www.ConciergeMedicineToday.com

"*I have to sell my practice. The [local insurance carrier] has taken the attack mode to my practice surrounding DPC. They sent letters to all my Patients that they will not recognize my license to practice medicine and will deny all referrals, claims and prescriptions.*"

- Family Medicine Doctor, New Hampshire

Working With Insurance Carriers.

How will transforming my practice into a Concierge Medicine, retainer, and membership medicine or DPC business model affect my current insurance contracts?

Doctors and medical practice administrators of a Concierge Medicine, retainer or DPC practice can choose for themselves whether or not they desire to participate in their local insurance carrier contracts.

Some concierge, retainer and DPC practices, however, do choose to continue participating in a smaller number of insurance plan contracts. The process for determining which insurance plans to continue accepting varies from office to office and state to state. Factors to consider in the determine participation may include:

- Concentration of Patients across contracted insurance carriers (i.e., payer mix);
- Favorable contract payment rates for primary care services;
- Timeliness of the plan's ability to process and pay out on a standing claim; and
- Value-added practice support services that are deemed advantageous to the practice.

For private-pay, (i.e. cash only) medical practices in states such as Alabama or Pennsylvania, many doctors elect to forgo insurance payment contracts entirely and operate solely off of their Patients' retainer fees and/or Patient fees collected at the time of service. One must be careful when doing so and understand their local marketplace. For example, if a large insurance carrier in your state provides health insurance for 97% of the population, such as the case in Alabama, opting out and terminating an insurance carrier contract could cause you to automatically be deemed as an out-of-network provider. This may not have a significant impact on your particular practice, depending upon the relationships you have established over the years with your Patients, but it does affect Patients who continue to have health insurance coverage, either through an employer-sponsored plan or an individual market plan.

The result is that insured Patients who choose to receive care through a Concierge Medicine, retainer-based or DPC practice may pay more out of pocket for primary care services. Many insurance carriers frown upon this termination of participation in their network due to the Patients who choose not to participate in the membership medicine program. For example, if a doctor has 3,000 Patients and elects to provide his/her Patients with Concierge Medicine healthcare services and does not want to accept or participate in insurance any longer, most of these doctors' offices will enroll between 125 to 600 Patients each. This then leaves the remaining 2,400-2,875 Patients in the local area looking for a primary care physician. While many Concierge Doctors' offices when they notify Patients help some Patients find another PCP in the area, insurance carriers are left to find and recruit more primary care doctors who will participate in their network and acquire these new Patients in an already strained and costly network.

According to surveys, interviews and online polls from over 1,000 Concierge Doctors across the U.S., over 80% of the currently operating Concierge Medicine or membership-based programs continue to accept insurance and participate in PPO and POS network contracts. For many doctors, participation in these network contracts is a safety net in the event the business model of Concierge Medicine they choose is flawed. The prospect of the possibility of suddenly losing 85%-95% all of their Patients in addition to terminating their long-held commercial insurance contracts is enough to cause a lot of doctors to have second thoughts about entering this marketplace.

"Many physicians do not seem to grasp the concept that there is a complete switch in revenue stream -- that the vast majority of their annual revenue is coming directly from annual fees," Roberta Greenspan, Founder of Specialdocs stated in an article to *MedScape* in July of 2013.

"The office fees that they bill to Medicare and commercial insurance, whether in or out of network, are really almost irrelevant. Of their entire annual income, maybe 15%-20% is office visit fees. And yet they panic."

The possibility of violating state insurance laws also gives rise to alarm. You cannot, for example, tell Patients that if they join your practice, they will no longer need insurance -- that for an annual fee, you will attend to all their medical needs. "That would mean that the physician himself is becoming a self-contained insurance provider. That is illegal in the lower 48 states," Greenspan warns.

The other thing that poses an issue is if the Patient is being enticed to join the concierge practice by being offered things that you wouldn't normally see in a medical practice, such as spa-like amenities or a nicer waiting room or transportation services, notes the MedScape article. Those could be considered payment for joining the practice and could be held under scrutiny under anti-kickback laws. In Greenspan's home state, Illinois, "the minute an Aetna or a Blue Cross or a United gets a whiff of the fact that any of our physicians in the Chicagoland area are 'going concierge,' they are out of the network immediately," she says. "They are just booted out. And that is something any commercial insurance company is privileged to do."

"One of the most difficult occurrences is when patients who does not understand the program or who philosophically disagrees with the membership fees (i.e. thinks this is for rich people) accuse the physician of abandoning them," says one former Transition Manager in Arizona. "Sometimes patients can be very vocal about their opinion of this and at times, be quite rude. This is very disheartening to most doctors, at least in the early stages of the transition process. 'Saying goodbye' to some long-term patients is one of the reasons many Physicians are reluctant to convert [to a Hybrid model]."

FAQs ...

From Patients About Insurance, Costs, Compatibility and Benefits of Concierge Medicine and DPC.

How Does Concierge Medicine and Some DPC Clinics Work With Health Insurance?

It is important to know and make clear in your communications to patients, both written and verbal that a fee paid to a Concierge Doctor is not considered in any way a type of insurance coverage, company or product. Payment to a Concierge Doctor in the form of a retainer or subscription fee entitles Patients to office-based services and telephone conferences if needed. (See Chapter 4 for Typical Services Provided).

Patients who are under the care of a Concierge Medicine physician are encouraged to be insured by a PPO, Medicare or a major medical plan. This allows for coverage of services provided outside of the doctor's office, such as catastrophic accidents, labs, radiology studies, specialty care and hospitalization.

Concierge Medicine Today discovered from 2009-2013, approximately 80% of Concierge Doctors' offices with annual and quarterly retainer fees, participate in Medicare or various PPO insurance plans. Medicare and other private insurances do not cover the annual fee.

The Direct Primary Care Journal in 2013-2014, interviewed and polled numerous DPC practices and found that approximately 40% of these offices participate of accept some form of insurance or participate in Medicare.

This is a completely separate fee that the Patient pays directly to the doctor or doctor's office in return for the enhanced access and other related services. Out-of-office charges and services provided by specialists and hospitalization expenses are billed directly to their insurance company or Medicare. Many Concierge Doctors' offices will bill the Patients insurance company or Medicare for services outside of the service contract the physician gives them when they sign up and pay the fee.

What About The Cost Of Prescription Medicines?

Oftentimes, a Concierge Doctor can start Patients out on treatment with samples. Beyond that, they and/or their insurance would be responsible. If they take several monthly prescriptions, they should contact their health insurance provider or consider a prescription discount program.

"When customer service is not the number one objective, members [i.e. Patients] will leave!"

-Mike Permenter, Industry Consultant

What if I need hospital services?

If a Patient has a life-threatening emergency, they should call 911.

Most concierge physicians retain admitting privileges at their local hospitals. If a concern or situation is not life-threatening, the Patient should contact their Concierge Physician directly. Most Concierge Doctors make themselves available to their Patients 24 hours a day for consultation. Should hospitalization be necessary, the concierge physician generally assists in coordinating their care during their stay. Specialty referrals can be discussed with the emergency room physician, if necessary and when a specialty consultation is needed, the Concierge Doctor typically knows who to recommend for sub-specialty care in your area.

Oftentimes, if the patient is hospitalized for an acute illness, a hospitalist physician will oversee their treatment until they are discharged to their regular concierge physician for follow-up care. Note that even when this is the case, a Concierge/DPC doctor should keep abreast of what is happening with the Patient. Making Patient contact or visiting the Patient while in the hospital goes a long way in cementing the doctor/patient relationship.

What Is The Retainer Or Subscription Fee?

The retainer or subscription fee is the fee paid by the Patient directly to the doctor for the enhanced services. Services vary depending upon the doctor, medical specialty, area and state. Fees may be paid on a monthly, quarterly, semi-annual or annual basis. However, most Concierge Doctors offer and detail a variety of services they provide to their Patients in the form of a 1 to 3 page Patient Agreement or sometimes called, a Member Services Agreement (MSA). The precise nature and scope of services to be provided at most Concierge Doctors' offices are set forth in this MSA, which is provided to the Patient upon request at virtually all Concierge Doctors' offices.

The MSA and the Concierge Doctor are not an insurance company or product. Most MSAs outline services based on more access with the doctor, so it is important for the Patient to review their health insurance coverage after they have joined a Concierge or DPC Doctors office to see whether a high-deductible health plan, HSA or FSA type of health insurance plan is more suitable for your personal needs.

In a 2014 interview with industry attorney, James Eischen, Esq., he tells *The Direct Primary Care Journal* ...

"Here are the basics: a) physicians, don't give tax advice to patients, tell them to consult their tax professional; b) the IRS regulations have found that a typical concierge annual fee is not an IRS Form 502 medical expense and therefore not suitable for HSA/FSA account payment; c) aspects of a private practice fee allocable to specific services or amenities (example: routine executive physical) could hypothetically qualify as a medical expense under Form 502, could be super-billed to the patient, and could justify the use of HSA/FSA funds (but

there are no regs or assurances from the IRS in this regard); and finally d) better not to ask how patients are paying or track the funds source—the reality is that the physician really does not want to be the gatekeeper on appropriate HSA/FSA funds use, and definitely does not want to deliver tax advice in that regard, ignorance is bliss in this regard. If the taxpayer's tax professional has studied the issue and advised the taxpayer that using the account is acceptable, the physician is not in a position to question or evaluate that advice, the physician lacks the relevant information and tax analysis. Any private medical practice that desires to maximize potential HSA/FSA patient funds use can do so by structuring the private medical practice in such a way as to avoid a "typical annual concierge annual fee" and allocate some (not all) of subscription fees to specific non-covered amenities that nonetheless qualify under Form 502 as "medical expenses." An attorney would be best involved."

Read more about this topic of DPC, Insurance, HDHP and HSAs at: www.DirectPrimaryCare.com – "HSA Center"

Concierge Medicine and DPC is all about access to the physician that the Patient may not have had before. Doctors recommend that their Patients obtain a high-deductible wraparound policy to cover catastrophic events and emergencies that may occur. Some efforts are underway, according to the California HealthCare Foundation report, stating ... 'To date, two insurance carriers have tailored offerings to direct care Patients, Cigna and Associated Mutual. Cigna has paired its "Level Pay" program targeting self-insured employers with 50-250 employees and is offering this only to certain customers at Qliance, based in Seattle, WA. Associated Mutual has stated it is offering a wraparound policy but hasn't announced details yet."

Can Patients Use Their Flexible Healthcare Spending Account To Cover The Cost Of A Concierge Doctor?

We would encourage Patients to check with their carrier or HR Department at their employer. Some Flex Accounts will allow them to use those pre-tax dollars to cover the annual fee.

Handling Medicare Issues

For many doctors, the appeal of Concierge Medicine is not having to deal with insurers. In an article to MedScape in July 2013, Specialdocs advises its Concierge Medicine physician clients to continue to take Medicare in addition to commercial insurance, if the insurer will allow it. In this business model, Patients pay an annual fee for an enhanced level of service and for non-covered services, such as wellness visits. Regular insurance takes care of the remaining covered services provided at the doctor's office.

Many Concierge Doctors who have chosen to walk into the legal minefield before you over the past 10-18 years who continue to accept insurance and also charge their Patients an additional fee for a higher level of service at their practice have run into legal problems in their state. Most Insurance Commissioner Offices have remained quiet on the issues surrounding

Concierge Medicine and a few have written formal statements stating the conclusion that this way of practicing medicine and treating Patients competes with local insurance carriers. If a physician collects a fee in advance for certain healthcare services, these Insurance Commission Offices say it can be considered pre-paid medical care, i.e. health insurance, and that this type of business practice will not be tolerated.

At present, these issues and others involving concierge medical care have been discussed in:

- 2009 Maryland Insurance Admin. Report: Report on "Retainer" or "Boutique" or "Concierge" Medical Practices and the Business of Insurance
- March 2006, West Virginia House bill 4021, Passed March 11, 2006
- 2005, GAO Report: Concierge Care Characteristics and Considerations for Medicare
- 2005, Massachusetts Senate Bill 1295
- 2004, Medicare Act, Section 605
- April 16, 2004, HMOs and the New York Department of Health Letter
- New Jersey Position on Concierge Medicine.
- More resources available for free – download at www.ConciergeMedicineToday.com

Handling Medicare Patients is a delicate subject. When a direct-pay, retainer or Concierge Medicine doctor chooses to opt-out of Medicare, they must continue to do so every two years. Let me explain. If you treat, visit or see any Medicare beneficiaries in your concierge medical practice, you must do one of these things: be enrolled as a Medicare provider, be a non-participating Medicare provider who is still subject to Medicare rules when treating Medicare Beneficiaries or, formally opt out of Medicare through your Medicare Administrative Contractor. If you do nothing you are considered a non-participating provider still subject to Medicare rules. You must file paperwork to opt-out of Medicare. It is at this point that you may privately contract with any Medicare Patients, so long as you are not billing Medicare for services you render.

Private contracting is an option for many Concierge Doctors and healthcare specialists like psychologists, who do not want to become Medicare providers but would like to furnish services to these beneficiaries. The primary difference between enrolled Medicare providers and those who furnish services through private contracts lies in how fees are collected. Medicare providers receive payment directly from Medicare, while those who opt out and privately contract with Patients collect payment directly from each Patient.

It is important to note that you cannot choose to opt out of Medicare for some beneficiaries but not others. It is an all-in or all-out decision you must make. If you do take Medicare as a concierge physician, you must be very careful to avoid duplicate billing for covered services. Doctors who are thinking about opting out of Medicare should consider whether beneficiaries would be able or willing to pay directly for your concierge medical, retainer or DPC healthcare and treatment services.

Annual physicals are typically a point of contention when talking about Concierge Medicine and retainer-based practices. The Accountable Care Act (ACA) now allows for annual physicals to be provided to Medicare recipients. For some Concierge Medicine offices, one of the largest attractions to an office is that comprehensive physicals are provided to Patients and included as part of the annual fee.

How do you differentiate between what a Medicare Patient will receive and what the Concierge Medicine member will get? Catherine Jordan, MSA, RN, LNCC, a legal nurse consultant who advises VantagePoint clients says "If it is not very carefully spelled out and then the Patient bills Medicare, Medicare pays for those services, and the physician accepts that payment, that physician can be charged with inappropriately billing Medicare for covered services and could be penalized and excluded from the Medicare program."

For Concierge Doctors to enter into private contracts with Medicare beneficiaries, physicians must file an affidavit with their Medicare Administrative Contractor (MAC) in their state and agree to not file any Medicare claims for a period of two years. Additionally, you must agree at this time to meet other certain criteria listed in the CMS web site pertaining to these beneficiaries. This affidavit must be refiled **every two years** in order for the health care professional to retain their opt-out status.

It is a little known fact that you must remember to opt out and notify your state's Medicare Administrative Contractor (MAC) every two years. If you opted out once it is not permanent. If two years passes without notifying your MAC at the end of the two year period, you are automatically enrolled as a Medicare provider again for another two years.

Concierge, DPC and retainer-based physician practices interested in privately contracting with Medicare beneficiaries should contact their MAC's provider enrollment department for more information about the opt out process and the CMS's requirements involved in private contracting. Some MACs have sample contract forms that providers may use or adapt in opting out of Medicare. Check with your local MAC provider enrollment department for guidance on how to contract privately with Medicare beneficiaries.

More information about <u>opting out and maintaining opt-out status</u> (PDF, 105KB) is available on the Regulations and Guidance section of the CMS website or visit: <u>http://www.cms.gov/Regulations-and-Guidance/Guidance/Transmittals/downloads/R92BP.pdf</u>.

True Story From Wisconsin
November 2013

After just six months, one physicians' DPC startup that bypassed the health insurance industry closed. The DPC doctor charged between $30 and $50 a month to provide primary care. He envisioned it to be very cost effective and designed it so it would work in combination with high-deductible insurance plans. By side-stepping the insurance industry, he told a local newspaper, he could operate his practice affordably because his time would be spent on Patients, not red tape.

In the email to Patients, the doctor explained that the Affordable Care Act presented 'insurmountable obstacles' for his practice to get a foothold in the local health care scene.

Concierge Medicine Today caught up with this entrepreneurial physician to get his side of the story.

"I wanted to try something different [entrepreneurial] and had over 100 Patients that were interested in the first two-months of startup. I was able to cover expenses with just 40 Patients." "Straight out of residency here, we have very few options and most involve working for an HMO in this area. The new sign-ups to the practice nearly stopped during the month of October, and people on the waiting list understandably wanted to remain there until the marketplace [i.e. Obamacare] was functioning more efficiently."

He also noted that other contributing factors to his closure included: personal obligations; the desire to make sound financial and business decisions; the ability to scale his DPC practice debt-free; and struggle to overcome objections and the uncertainty of prospective Patients related to the Affordable Care Act; and others.

"The Affordable Care Act marketplace presented a lot of problems for my practice," the article noted. "This is ironic, since a more transparent marketplace would be beneficial for me, but I did not foresee a broken website, a government shutdown and more expensive insurance for many of my Patients. The new signups to the practice nearly stopped during the month of October, and people on the waiting list understandably wanted to remain there until the marketplace was functioning. This still hasn't happened."

"We all saw this coming and chose to a large extent to ignore it. Extended hours, a simple, surefire way to expand a client/Patient base is slow in coming. Who works 9-5 anymore? If our Patients do not, why do we? At what point do we choose a walk-in-clinic over trekking all over town for all the tests our doctor ordered? In a perfect world (circa 1982) your primary care physician knew your family from cradle into adulthood and beyond. If we choose to be client focused we might be surprised at the rate of growth and influx of Patients – why do not we give it a try?"

-Esther, EBA Consulting

If a concierge, DPC or retainer physician practice chooses to continue participating in a chosen list of insurance plan contracts, the practice must make it very clear to Patients what healthcare treatments, medical services and procedures are going to be covered by the insurance carrier contract. Most insurance plans and carriers will not pay for services determined to be covered by the Patients existing health insurance plan, Medicare or the retainer fee that the physician has set-up.

Do You Have Additional Legal or Insurance Carrier Concerns?

The regulations governing the development of a Concierge Medicine, boutique, retainer, or DPC practice vary from state to state. You should contact your legal counsel in order to assure compliance with local insurance and state regulations.

Recommended Reading

AMA Issues Ethical Standards Related To Retainer-Style Practices.

For a copy of the AMA's guidelines for concierge practices, visit www.ama-assn.org
or contact the

Council on Ethical and Judicial Affairs,
American Medical Assn.
515 N. State Street
Chicago, IL 60610;

Tel: 312-464-4823
Fax: 312-464-4799
E-mail: ceja@ama-assn.org

Also available at: www.ConciergeMedicineToday.com

Recommended Reading

AAFP Statement On DPC (DPC)

For a copy of the AAFP's statement on DPC practices, visit www.aafp.org
or
download a copy at: www.ConciergeMedicineToday.com

"The conversion process is not an easy one."

-Jeffrey S. Gorodetsky, M.D., Stuart, FL

Move With A Plan.

Starting Your Concierge Medicine or DPC Practice Right: Service Offering Planning and Identification.

The journey is more fun if you know where you are going.

If you are one of the thousands of physicians, emergency room doctors or recent medical school graduates currently considering starting up a DPC or Concierge Medicine practice, the first thing you need to seriously consider is not your start-up budget, not the location and not the hours you will be working. The first thing you must consider are the services you will be selling and the business model you want to use. The old adage holds true, 'Plan your work – then work your Plan.' Patients, start-up capital, leased space and even employees will follow a confident leader with a plan.

Doctors today considering entering this niche marketplace must understand that doing good work by caring for the Patient isn't the whole job. Part of 'getting there' (the job you dream of), is that things like the unique services you incorporate into your physician-Patient contract actually matter — even when you do not think they will. My favorite story to write is from the physician who transitioned in the past two or three years and says 'I wish I had done this years ago.'

In putting legs to this concept, make sure you understand the services you plan on offering to your Patients and local community before making financial business and emotional decisions on everything else. Remember, your major investment will obviously be in the purchase of the leased office space itself. It usually runs over 60% of the Concierge Medicine and DPC clinics budget, according to *The Concierge Medicine Research Collective*, 2013. However, the type of services you will be offering and selling will determine the type of office you are going to need.

Based upon countless interviews with doctors is that one of the first things doctors do when they start a Concierge Medicine or DPC practice is to reduce the number of leased office space they use and the amount of employees they have. Most offices average between 1-2 employees according to *Concierge Medicine Today*. So, research which type of office space are most used for provided the services you are basing your new medical practice upon. This will serve to narrow down the list of equipment and operational components to something that is much more manageable and functional for you and future staff.

Next, what can you offer that is something unique and new for your Patients? A coffee or beverage bar in your lobby area? A flat screen cable TV? Screensavers on tablet devices in the exam rooms promoting a new service or device you are using in your practice? Do they need a place to sit down and take some rest time. After all, they are probably seeing you because they need a short time out. Just because this is a Concierge Medicine or DPC operation does not mean you forget about adding value for Patients. Renewal rates at a number of concierge medical clinics nationwide are declining because physicians are over-promising and under-delivering services to their Patients. What strategies are you going to implement to help differentiate you from the rest of the competition and keep your patients feeling cared for and special?

Service Selection

Office space you will need to consider is the volume of Patients you are going to be seeing on a daily basis. Most Concierge Medicine clinics see an average of 5 to 10 Patients per day, according to *Concierge Medicine Today*. This will affect how many employees you are going to need in the practice to assist with administrative support, sales, blood pressure checks, etc., and this, in turn, will impact the actual space needed for your front office. If it is too small, you may lose sales and valuable Patients; too large and you waste valuable investment capital.

Common Service Menu

Some Of The Most Common Services Include:

- Doctor On Call 24/7
- House Calls
- No Waiting
- Same Day Appointments
- Unlimited Appointments For Your Membership Fee
- "Executive physical exams" that may include a full body scan, screening for 200 diseases, blood tests for rare conditions and time spent with the physician going over every aspect of the Patients medical history.
- Routine Lab Tests
- X-rays
- Coordination Of Care If A Patient Becomes Ill While Traveling
- Mental Health Services
- Well-Baby Checks (Offered At Some Family Medicine Offices)
- Online Access To Medical Records
- Home Delivery Of Medications
- Hospital Visits From The Doctor
- Transportation To Appointments
- Coordinated Care With Specialists During Travel
- Hotel Reservations For Family During A Medical Crisis
- Wellness, Fitness And Lifestyle Screenings
- Weight Management Counseling
- Nutritional Counseling
- Health Strategy

Please note, each and every doctor should decide what services are included in their practice membership(s). These are only examples of some of the common services offered. Your practice and membership may or may not include some or all of these types of services.

A Poll Conducted By *Concierge Medicine Today* In 2013 Found That:
The Concierge Medicine Research Collective, ConciergeMedicineToday.com

- 74% | Yes. We include home visits to our Patients as needed.

- 26% | No. We do not include home visits as part of the Patient-physician agreement.

Lastly, consider how you will incorporate technology, cell phone visits, SMS text messaging, appointment reminders and local or home visits into your practice timescales. When will you rollout home visits? How soon will you implement credit card statements? Between acquiring the basic operational technology for your new startup practice and the time it takes to acquire a new Patient sizeable investment in this new venture.

In closing, Concierge Medicine and DPC is all about the Patient — offering something of value with price transparency and affordability. The more planning you place on your services now before you begin, the greater your success will be in the very near future.

"Shortly after I opened my concierge practice in Prescott one of my new Patients said ... 'I really like coming to your office because I do not feel like I am at Disneyland.' I was perplexed by his statement and asked him, 'What do you mean?' He replied, 'It is not a three hour wait and a 20 second ride like it is when I take the kids to Disneyland.'

-Eugene T. Conte, D.O. FAOCD
Prescott, AZ | Cosmetic Dermatology Associates of Prescott*

Choose The Business Model Right For Your Local Marketplace.

The 3 Most Common Business Models Used Today.

The Fee For Non-Covered Services Model (FNCS)

Many doctors have chosen to partner with large franchise Concierge Medicine businesses to help with the startup and transition needs necessary to open their Concierge Medicine or DPC practice. However, more than half of all concierge physicians have opted to use accountants, attorneys, practice managers and business consultants to navigate their way into the new practice model. As more and more doctors begin to analyze and potentially move into concierge medical practices, independent physicians are choosing not to be a part of a large franchise operation and instead are transitioning with a smaller consultant. The Doctor should examine their fee structure and price their services competitively.

"I perform a thorough analysis of the practice and determine areas where expenses will be reduced," said Mike Permenter, a private consultant specializing in DPC models. "After a survey of the physician's Patients, we conduct a 12-18 week conversion. Our fees are collected during the transition only. Once a successful conversion has been completed, we help train the physician staff to provide membership services. If customer service is maintained, we know the practice will continue growing without a need for further services."

Most doctors currently practicing Concierge Medicine as a career choice fall into one of two intelligence-gathering categories when they first opened. First, they used a franchise concierge company to help them with the details or they opted to do it themselves and surround themselves with a local team that would provide counsel in starting this practice model.

Over the past four years Concierge Doctors operating under the direction of a large franchise concierge company or consultancy will price services, on average, between $1,200 and $1,800 per Patient and opening with a Patient load between 300-750 Patients. This helps the practice compete with local retail clinics, pharmacy chains, and primary care doc-in-a-box practices and attracts, en masse, the demographic that practice needs in order to succeed in their local market. They also learned that many independent Concierge Doctors who chose not to operate under the guidance of a franchise business model were charging much more for their services, between $2,500 – $5,000 per Patient, and opening with a Patient load of 75-180 Patients under their care.

The premise of most franchise Concierge Medicine business models, termed "Fee For Non-Covered Services Model," reduces the size of a medical practice to a more manageable Patient load and these Patients agree to pay a fee for more time with their physician, an annual physical, and more personalized access and service. Emphasis is on a healthier lifestyle, both for the members and the physician. According to a national poll of Concierge Doctors from 2010-2012 by *Concierge Medicine Today*, approximately 80% of these practices accept most major insurance plans and participate in Medicare. The "Fee For Non-Covered Services Model" allows for Medicare and private insurance to be billed by the physician for routine visits and procedures. To date, this model comprises the largest segment of the market, approximately 46 states, although DPC (Fee For Care Model), is rapidly catching up in select markets.

Distinct Advantages For Selecting The "FNCS" Model Include:

Physicians who are looking to slow down without affecting their current income levels will find this model attractive. These types of models offer an enhanced physical (or some enhanced procedure or procedures not covered by Medicare), on an annual basis, which is the basis for the entire fee. Fees for these models usually range from $1,200 – $2,000. It is critical that physicians converting to this business model are able to **reduce expenses** to accommodate this type of practice.

There are typically a maximum number of Patients allowed to join the practice, usually around 600. Industry sources tell *Concierge Medicine Today* that they have not seen too many of these Concierge Medicine practices reach the 600 Patient-member levels, but that most are satisfied at the 400 Patient-member levels.

Contrary to what people think, this model is **not** just for the rich as the vast majority of Patients make less than $100K, according to industry surveys. The Concierge Medicine industry has been touted by the media and television for years as an expensive way to see the doctor that you have known for years. At the inception of the movement in the early to mid-'90's, this was factually true. What is not truthful is that nearly two decades later, the majority of Concierge Medicine and DPC offices cost their Patients between $50 – $135 per month.

Most Family Practice Doctors typically offer a family plan where dependent children up to a certain age are covered free. Internal Medicine Physicians may offer a similar program but typically for dependent children between the ages of 16 and 25. Therefore there are many single moms joining these practices.

There are many development teams and implementation companies that are helping doctors to convert to these more price transparent business models. They, for the most part, have every base covered in regard to ensuring a successful launch. There is a very high failure rate for doctors trying to transition to this type of model on their own. The conversion process is intense and every transition has its own unique challenges.

Distinct Disadvantages For Selecting The "FNCS" Model Are:

The FNCS business model works very well when implemented appropriately. Although a medical practice is considerably smaller and much easier to manage, there are still existing issues with regards to billing Medicare and insurance companies, collecting co-pays, checking Patients in and out, etc. This not only increases operational costs, but most of the problems surround billing insurance. Alternatively, in other concierge and direct primary business models, operational costs are much lower because the physicians/practice do not participate in Medicare or insurance plans.

FNCS Business Models require that the services paid for by members are not Medicare covered services. Accordingly, it is critical to have legal input with regard to structuring this model. Because Medicare regulations are likely to change frequently, especially with the ACA, ongoing legal monitoring is necessary in this type of model.

According to a recent 2013 *Physicians Practice* Survey respondents in practices of six-to-10 physicians reported practicing in a concierge/membership practice. Here are some more specific findings from the survey:

- *Solo practices: 2 percent are in concierge/membership practices.*
- *Two- to five-physician practices: 2 percent are in concierge/membership practices.*
- *Six- to 10-physician practices: 5 percent are in concierge/membership practices.*
- *11- to 20-physician practices: No respondents are concierge/membership practices.*
- *20-plus physician practices: 1 percent of respondents are concierge/membership practices.*

It is likely that more doctors, especially doctors in smaller practices, will begin transitioning to concierge, membership, and DPC in the coming years. Physicians who favor independent practice will likely view these alternative reimbursement models as a way to retain their independence, spend more time with Patients, and combat declining reimbursement.

"Instead of viewing the status quo PCP model as the center of the universe. Maybe we should take some plays from the Retail Clinic playbook before we become obsolete."

~Dr. Robert Nelson, DPC Physician, MyDocPPS.com Cumming, GA.

Hybrid Or Segmented Model:

The business and day-to-day operation of any medical practice is challenging. Concierge and Direct Practice doctors will tell you the same challenges exist in their business model as well. Some physicians are operating their medical practices in what is called a "Hybrid" or "Segmented" business model. "Hybrid" Concierge Medicine practice is where physicians charge a monthly, quarterly or annual retainer or membership fee for services for which Medicare and insurers do not pay. Under this model, practices and physicians will bill Medicare and insurance companies for Patient visits and covered by the plans. They also offer a traditional model of healthcare which is generally staffed by a Nurse Practitioner (NP) or a Physician's Assistant (PA). These two levels of service are offered under the same roof but have very different payment models.

What Does This Look Like Practically?

Simply stated, the medical practice has two businesses under one roof, Business 'A' and Business 'B.' Under Business 'A' those Patients wishing to be treated by the doctor will likely pay a monthly, quarterly or annual fee to the practice and receive services such as: quick appointments; email access; phone consultations; newsletters; an annual physical, prolonged visits and comprehensive wellness and health strategy plans. Business 'A' will bill Medicare and the Patients' insurance company for visits and services covered. Business 'B' however, is where the Patients schedule an appointment to see a Nurse Practitioner or a PA and that care is overseen by the doctor in the practice. Business 'B' will bill Medicare and the Patient's insurance company for visits and services covered by the plan, accept co-pays, deductibles, etc. If Patients on Side 'B' must see the overseeing doctor, it is very likely they will see them.

So Why Join Business 'A' of the Physician's Practice?

As stated above, services inside a "Hybrid" Concierge Medicine practice on Business 'A' are likely to include: quick appointments; email access; phone consultations; newsletters; annual physical, prolonged visits and comprehensive wellness and health strategy plans. These services, along with ensuring they will maintain an ongoing relationship with their Physician, are very attractive to some Patients, and they are willing to pay for it. Patients should check with their Doctor to find out what services are included in their Membership Service Agreement (MSA). These are only examples of some of the typical services provided. Services vary by state, physician and specialty.

Advantages To Physicians Operating Under The "Hybrid" Concierge Medicine Practice Model

- Physicians who operate in a "hybrid" Concierge Medicine business model typically see 10 Patients per day.

- Allows the Doctor to continue participation in Patients' health plans and Medicare. According to *Concierge Medicine Today*, over 80% of Concierge Medicine practices in the U.S. do so.
- Spend more than 30-minutes per visit with each of their Patients, allowing doctors to get to know their Patients better, and investigate symptoms and lifestyle habits more closely.
- Increased annual reimbursement compared to traditional, managed care and insurance-driven primary care practices.
- More time to research valuable, cost saving treatment options and drugs for your Patients.
- Provides a safety net for you in the transition process as this dual model approach initially has less disenfranchised Patients and less stress and anxiety throughout the transition process as Patients continue to participate in the insured, non-concierge side of your practice.
- More time to spend with your family.

The "Hybrid" Challenge

Such as in life, nothing good ever comes easy. The transition to a "Hybrid" Concierge Medicine model or "Fee-for-Non-Covered-Services Model" has its challenges. When a physician chooses the "Hybrid" business model, he/she must first carefully interview either a Physician Assistant (PA), a Nurse Practitioner (NP) or Physician partner that will replace you and your time under Business 'B' of the practice while you migrate and start Business 'A.' Most physicians hire a PA or NP for cost reasons. Once this is accomplished, a physician needs to spend some time explaining reasons why he is opening up Business 'A' of his practice and taking on a more formal 'observational' role of Business 'B' of the practice.

Sometimes, transition consultants who assist doctors in establishing a "Hybrid" concierge medical practice will train a temporary transition manager whose job it is to mirror the physician's schedule. That Transition Manager available to meet with Patients as they come through the office on their regular visits, explain the benefits of joining Business 'A' of the practice and what the cost, features and benefits are. All the while, informing Patients that they can still come to this location and see an NP or PA for their regular care, if they choose to do so and not join Business 'A'.

"One of the most difficult occurrences is when Patients who do not understand the program or who philosophically disagree with the membership fees (i.e. thinks this is for rich people) accuse the physician of abandoning them," says one former Transition Manager in Arizona. "Sometimes Patients can be very vocal about their opinion of this and at times, be quite rude. This is very disheartening to most doctors, at least in the early stages of the transition process. 'Saying goodbye' to some long-term Patients is one of the reasons many Physicians are reluctant to convert [to a Hybrid model]."

There are some distinct implementation and management challenges to the "Hybrid" model. Physicians are strongly encouraged to establish a team of trusted advisors, which may include:

- a "Hybrid" medical practice consultant;
- a Transition Manager;
- an Attorney;
- a supportive spouse;
- and an Accountant ... to name a few.

"Patients are educated, possibly more than ever, as a result of the changes to our healthcare system," adds Richard Doughty, CEO of Cypress Concierge Medicine based in Louisiana. "Patients are looking for answers and options and taking more initiative in their overall health. Following their doctor into Concierge Medicine for many Patients is exactly the vehicle that meets their needs. In addition, knowing others who have benefitted from that relationship with their Concierge Doctor confirms the value as their doctor makes this change."

Some of the other challenges to overcome include:

The average membership is typically much lower than other models because Patients are given the option to stay with the practice, as they always have, but to see a PA or NP under their insurance. Patients understand that the NP or the PA has to be overseen by the Doctor and if they need their doctor, it is likely they will request to and be able to see him/her.

There are great NPs and PAs. But not many of them will jump on the doctor's hamster wheel and see 30 to 40 Patients per day. Especially when they see their overseeing physician treat 6-10 Patients per day. There is likely to be high turnover of NPs and PAs as well as burnout among staff and other support members. Frequently the Physician will decide to work both sides of the practice in order to help the NP or PA. Once this occurs, Concierge members have been known to leave the "A" side of the practice as they see no differentiation, or at least not enough to pay a fee.

The staff that is helping the NP or PA is as busy trying to manage the chaos as they have been in the past. Support staff is crucial to highlighting the doctors Business 'A' of the practice. Customer service is key. There is likely to be high turnover among these team members. If you share staff, this can create its own set of dilemmas. If part of the time some staff are frantically moving Patients through Business 'B' of the practice to see the PA or NP and then are relied upon to switch hats and be a strong advocate and customer service representative to the 'A' side, some Patients and things are going to be mismanaged and forgotten. This message, that there really is no difference, will ultimately be communicated to Patients on both sides of the practice. If there is a lack of customer service Patients have been found to leave the practice entirely.

The most important challenge to the model is trying to keep it profitable. Typically, in addition to a lower number of members, there is also a significant number of Patients that will leave the practice altogether, choosing not to participate in either Business 'A' or Business 'B.'

Frequently, the doctor believes that his/her membership fees produce additional revenues added to the revenue of his/her original practice, and that he/she is likely to earn $300k – $500k more with this type of business model. In addition, since there are no decreases in the size of the overall practice, and Business 'B' of the practice requires billing support, it is very difficult to reduce expenses in these types of "hybrid" concierge medical business models.

"With the right planning, a hybrid can be converted to a DPC model," says Mike Permenter, industry expert and consultant to physicians. "I predict there will be many hybrids converting to a DPC model in the future."

MDVIP, the country's largest concierge medical group, has contracts with around 700+ practices and operates in nearly every state across the contiguous U.S. They have been operating and helping physicians enter into Concierge Medicine business models for over a decade.

"When I first heard about hybrid type models I was excited about a model that would allow some of the Patients to become members of the concierge side of the practice while the rest were seen by a mid-level Nurse Practitioner or Physician's Assistant." notes Permenter. "After all, this would eliminate having to part with those long-term Patients. They could just remain in the practice and see the mid-level, and their insurance would be billed as always. It turned out not to be so attractive for both the Patients and the Physician" in Permenter's opinion.

All in all, "Hybrid" Concierge Medicine programs can be successful if the transition is done appropriately. There are a few companies that specialize in these transitions. We have a list of those companies on www.ConciergeMedicineToday.com or you may email us at editor@conciergemedicinetoday.com.

The Fee For Care (FFC) or DPC (DPC) Model:
Pros And Cons Of Operating A DPC Practice (DPC)

There is a third model commonly referred to as DPC or a Fee For Care (FFC) type of practice. The California Healthcare Foundation describes DPC as an emerging model that has gained some attention in California and nationally in recent years. Sometimes referred to as "retainer practices," DPC practices generally do not accept health insurance, instead serving Patients in exchange for a recurring monthly fee — usually $50 to $100 — for a defined set of medical services.

Source: http://www.chcf.org/publications/2013/04/retainer-direct-primary-care#ixzz2ru8Mh8N3

The practice generally does not bill insurance and charges Patients fees for treatment and care under the price point of $100 per month. Some prices are age-banded and have been found to treat children in this type of practice for under $10 per month.

"20 to 25 DPC Doctors can take care of 20K patients," said Dr. Garrison Bliss, Founder of Qliance based in Seattle, WA in a recent 2014 interview with *The Direct Primary Care Journal*. "This is a reflection of the enormous need for high functioning primary care in the US. In a DPC world, the doctor and the patient govern that world because nobody else can. Working for larger numbers of patients and working for larger companies and institutions is fraught with big challenges, but the culture of DPC appears to be strong enough to withstand those challenges."

"Having access to a care provider with the time to provide the care is key, and growth at this pace makes it hard to stay ahead of the demand – but we have already demonstrated that the quality of the care and the patient experience is miles ahead of the existing primary care structures. We dramatically reduce the cost of care while improving the access to care for populations like Medicaid and Insurance Exchange patients in Washington State – something that I had hoped to see but could only dream about until the last year. When stable at scale, organizations like Qliance can demonstrate the power of relationship, service, patient empowerment and freedom from insurance fee-for-service incentives to reorient and support primary care in a way that has already surprised many of us from within the movement. Someone has to stand up and volunteer to care for America. If not DPC, then who?"

Qliance, MedLion and other emerging companies have popularized this offshoot of the Concierge Medicine business model. Additionally, five large practice organizations that use the membership model are listed below. The Patient rosters are estimations:

- Paladina Health, with 8,000+ Patients
- Qliance, with 40k+ Patients
- Iora Health, with 2,400+ Patients
- MedLion, with 3,000+ Patients
- White Glove Health, with 40,000+ Patients via self-insured employers and 450,000 via health plans

DPC providers help keep costs low by avoiding unnecessary referrals and by referring mainly to specialists willing to offer significant discounts. Despite this advantage, the DPC model may be hampered by a lack of awareness health plans and primary care physicians, resistance from some insurers, and resistance from competing hospitals and specialists.

DPC medical clinics and doctors with price points under $100 per person per month are slowly gaining traction in the highly competitive healthcare marketplace across the U.S. Their strength has not been in the number of physicians signing up to change their business model but in the

In addition, physicians now working in this space according to *The DPC Journal* are between 100-200 doctors nationwide and growing.

As one of the world's leading online travel companies, Expedia, Inc. (EXPE) knows not to under-estimate the power of a good vacation on improving one's state of mind. So when the company realized a few years ago that a majority of its workforce was not using their fully-allotted vacation time, business leaders saw a need to practice what they preach. In addition to implementing a revised vacation policy, Expedia, Inc. also elected to begin offering an annual travel allowance to help fund employees' vacation travel during their downtime.

The company recently partnered with Qliance, a leading healthcare organization operating a network of clinics that provide comprehensive primary and its preventive care services, to open an onsite clinic at its Bellevue, Washington headquarters. Now, Expedia, Inc. employees and their dependents have easy access to primary health care services, including Saturday hours. The company hopes this effort will help prevent treatable symptoms from becoming chronic issues and encourage employees to use their sick time and medical benefits when needed. In just the first month of operation, employees and their dependents utilized nearly 300 office visits at the clinic.

"We are really pleased at how much use the clinic has received so far," said Connie Symes, Executive Vice President of Human Resources at Expedia, Inc. "It is great to see that the tools being provided are making health and well-being more convenient and accessible. As an employer, we spend a great deal of time attracting the best and brightest talent and we are equally focused on helping them be active and engaged employees of Expedia, Inc. We have a vested stake in the vitality of our workforce, and so we really cannot afford not to make preventative care a top priority for our employees."

"One of the things I encourage [DPC] doctors do during their first couple of years in this new delivery model is give yourself a raise. This encourages you emotionally and helps builds your confidence."

~Dr. Chris Ewin, a DPC Doctor at 121MD in Dallas, TX in an interview with The Direct Primary Care Journal, October 2014. "

Consulting companies from the Concierge Medicine marketplace are also helping struggling physicians move into the DPC space. These companies are helping physicians discontinue their relationships with most, if not all, insurance and seeking agreements with employers in the doctor's local community. They couple those self-insured health plan programs with a primary care (i.e. DPC) physician. Typically this is accomplished when a high deductible insurance plan and/or a supplement plan can cover a Patient's deductible. Many physicians are finding that annual or monthly fees for their Patients are being paid for by the employers They have partnered with.

While the business models are still evolving, most DPC medical practice models require that the doctor opt-out of Medicare and insurance.

As most DPC physicians today will tell you, you can adjust your prices according to your particular area but you should develop a comprehensive primary care treatment model that can encompass your membership fee. Each physician should determine the size of the panel and the annual membership fee by developing a pro-forma, outlining services, overhead costs and salaries. The success of most DPC and Concierge Medicine models is mostly attributed to how well the doctor and the practice provide high-touch, quality customer service. If this philosophy is carried out throughout the practice, with the staff and inherently part of your office culture, your DPC practice will grow, renewal rates will be high and Patient referrals will be your reward for a job well done.

As a word of caution, Mike Permenter, industry expert and physician consultant says "the only downside to this model is the allure to keep increasing the Patient panel size, therefore damaging customer service. However, for the first time physicians can look at their practice as a business. If memberships are tied to employee benefits, it is possible for one or two good companies to produce enough members to support more than one practice, opening the door for multi-practice suites where even young physicians can be recruited to step right into a DPC practice with a full Patient Panel."

Rob Lamberts, MD, a DPC physician from Augusta, GA writes ...

"I am now up to nearly 400 Patients, and while we have talked about hiring a new staff person, we seem to be hitting our stride in this different practice model and have not yet been overwhelmed. New Patients are coming with regularity, some still coming from my old practice and many others through word-of-mouth from satisfied Patients. Yes, people still seem very satisfied with the care they are getting from me. If they have medical problems that need immediate attention, they can come in and be seen. I frequently hear from Patients in the office how happy they are that I am doing this kind of practice.

I have also stepped up my effort to coordinate care by calling specialists or sending them detailed letters explaining why I need them to see the Patient. The specialists I have contacted are delighted with my efforts to make their jobs easier and to give better care. While it is still difficult to get them to adopt secure communication tools, I am getting a small number who I can throw curbside consults to, and who can give me updates on the Patients from their computers or phones.

I have been working on adding new services as well. One of the first things I did when I opened the office was to negotiate a very inexpensive fee schedule from a lab that would bill me for the tests. Most docs mark up the tests and make a profit off of it, but I do very little mark-up of the tests, instead offering things like a CBC for $4.50 and a TSH for $8.00. I am now working on doing the same thing with an x-ray facility, giving them the opportunity to get guaranteed cash up-front (reducing their overhead) while avoiding the many traps of compliance with Medicare billing (which forbids providers from giving discounts to other Patients that they do not give to Medicare Patients)."

"I can attest: get into the cash-pay world and life becomes simpler and overhead is much, much lower. You can afford much cheaper rates. In the end, I hope to negotiate this kind of rate for other procedures, like echocardiograms, colonoscopies, and perhaps even minor surgeries. As my Patient population grows, my credibility in negotiation grows as well."

-Rob Lamberts, MD, DPC Physician from Augusta, GA

The transition into a DPC model is very similar to Concierge Medicine, industry consultants say. Every prospective Patient (i.e. member) needs to understand that even though the physician is not billing insurance, they can still participate in the practice. Further, that their membership fees, which pay for their primary care, will result in overall savings for the member.

"At the beginning of 2013 I stared into the great unknown of this new practice," says Dr. Lamberts. "I had no idea which plans would succeed and which were foolish dreams. The road was much more difficult than I expected, but also much more satisfying. I spent much of my time learning what does not work, but in the end learned that most good ideas grow out of the remains of a hundred bad ones that didn't survive."

"Now, as I face 2014 I see great opportunity. My dreams are still big; I am more convinced than ever that this model of practice could be a game changer for American health care. But my ambitions have grown smaller. I now enjoy the practice of medicine more than I have in many years, and am delighted by the same expression on the faces of my Patients. It does not suck to be a doctor anymore, and it does not suck for my Patients to go to the doctor! My ambition is to keep that reality alive for me while making it available for more Patients. I want them to be happy, and I want to be happy. It is nice to think it actually could be a happy new year."

As with any business, appropriate legal insight is necessary when considering a fee adjustment, particularly when it comes to healthcare, dealing with Patients, communicating with insurers, etc. All agreements between the DPC practice and the Patient(s) and employer in your local area should be carefully examined by a trusted healthcare attorney specializing in health law and healthcare matters. Your tax attorney probably is not the only attorney you should be talking to if you are considering a future in either DPC or Concierge Medicine.

The DPC Medical Practice Cons:

To date, Patients of healthcare relate DPC, retail medicine, Concierge Doctors and the convenient care clinics to be cash-only healthcare. The masses in America do not yet understand the many features and benefits of these practices and that they are manned primarily by primary care physicians. This low, brand exposure coupled with the fact that many primary care practices are selling out to large health systems, is creating unfavorable economic conditions for DPC to grow.

Many DPC practices are small, individual practices. As of late, there are not enough (less than 400 according to estimates by *The DPC Journal*, 2014), to service large, national employer groups. Beta tests in Seattle, WA between practices like Qliance and companies such as Expedia, Inc., however, are currently being watched carefully. Today Qliance operates five clinics in Washington. The largest is in Seattle, which employs six full-time doctors and a nurse. As of 2011, there are 24 direct primary care practices in the state serving 10,525 patients.

Most DPC practices have reduced the amount of office square footage from an average of 5,000 SF to roughly 2,500 SF. Last, because Medicare billing and insurance billing is almost nonexistent, the need for a billing department and administrative overhead is nearly gone. Industry consultants find that many times, the doctor is reluctant to reduce staff that has been a part of the practice for a long time but that this is a business decision that has to be considered if doctors are considering a future in DPC.

Concierge Medicine and DPC is not comprehensive and not considered insurance care. It is all about access to the physician that Patients did not have before. Doctors should recommend that their Patients obtain a high-deductible wraparound policy to cover catastrophic events and emergencies that may occur. Some efforts are underway according to the California HealthCare Foundation report, published earlier this year stating ... 'To date, two insurance carriers have tailored offerings to direct care Patients, Cigna and Associated Mutual. Cigna has paired its "Level Pay" program targeting self-insured employers with 50-250 employees and is offering this only to certain customers at Qliance, based in Seattle, WA.

UPDATE: From ACO News: "Qliance amasses 20,000 patients," Jan. 6, 2014

By Kristin Sims-Kastelein January 6, 2014 [PUGET SOUND, Wash.]— New business growth under the Health Insurance Marketplace and growth within existing business segments has led Qliance, a concierge primary care model for the masses, to care for 20,000 people in the Puget Sound area. In six and a half years, the privately held company has grown from one clinic to five and employs 14 primary care doctors. Its goal is to bring high quality, service intense primary care to Americans, while bringing down the total cost of health care.

READ FULL STORY ... Source: http://www.accountablecaremedia.com/qliance-amasses-20000-patients-company-provides-boutique-primary-care-for-the-masses/

UPDATE! Qliance is an option in the Exchange under the Coordinated Care 'ambetter' Health Plan for Individuals. (Source: http://directprimarycare.wordpress.com/2014/07/06/qliance-is-an-option-in-the-exchange-under-the-coordinated-care-ambetter-health-plan-for-individuals/)

Many DPC physicians opt to keep their monthly, per Patient fee between $50-$100 because of its appeal to a larger segment of the population which increases revenue. Since this low fee is so attractive to so many people, one of the greatest downfalls of a DPC practice model is the ability to 'promise-and-deliver' to those Patients/members that you have brought into the practice. Meaning, you may not be able to any longer provide same-day appointments and 30-minute appointments because you now have a primary care Patient panel of 1,500 members. A critical component to the success and attractive benefits of DPC to a Patient population is the high-touch, quality time, same-day, no-wait, no-hassle access to a doctor. Physicians have to analyze carefully their pricing prior to launch and be sure that they can offer outstanding customer service at that price point. Pricing your practice too low and filtering most of your Patients to a PA or RN at the practice will hurt Patient renewals in the long-run. A doctor should at all times ensure that there is an appropriate ratio of Patients-to-physicians at all times.

The DPC Medical Practice Pros:

Many people are unaware that there was a clause was written into the ACA allowing retainer practices to be included in the proposed insurance exchanges – with the caveat that these practices be paired with a wraparound insurance policy covering services outside of primary care. According to a report by The California HealthCare Foundation, It is the only non-insurance offering to be authorized in the insurance exchanges slated to begin in 2014; however there is not a specific requirement that DPC be included.

Due to much smaller Patient panels than traditional primary care and insurance-based medical practices, DPC doctors say they spend more time with Patients, discussing treatments, procedures, prescription use and other healthcare options. Similar to its older familial medical model, Concierge Medicine, DPC doctors frequently promote the fact that they can provide "unhurried appointments" and same-day access to a physician.

Significant venture capital dollars coupled with employer interest in certain metropolitan areas across the U.S. have helped advance practice models like Qliance in Seattle, WA. This financial backing plus the interest from large insurance companies to beta-test wrap around insurance products with these types of physicians has also helped DPC to prove its viability in the marketplace over the past several years.

Update! Effective January 1, 2015, applicable large employers with 50+ full-time equivalent (FTE) employees without minimum essential health care coverage could be assessed a penalty. Offering Qliance with current benefits plans provides employees quality care while saving companies money.

The ability to create a medical practice whereby one physician can opt out of Medicare and discontinue insurance billing allows the practice to reduce overhead expenses significantly.

Physicians have worked closely over the past few years with business experts and accountants to help forecast what their net revenue will be under this financial business model. Because DPC and Concierge Medicine are some of the only medical business models in healthcare that allow a physician to more accurately forecast what they will 'net' at the end of each year, makes these business models appealing to doctors.

"One of the things I encourage [DPC] doctors do during their first couple of years in this new delivery model is give yourself a raise," says Dr. Chris Ewin, a DPC Doctor in Dallas, TX in an interview with *The Direct Primary Care Journal*, October 2014. "This encourages you emotionally and helps builds your confidence."

Meanwhile, while creating these financial preforms, doctors have been able to develop membership and program options for their Patients that can meet the needs of just about every income demographic. One doctor might charge $20,000 per year and only want 150 Patients, while another physician may charge $95.00 per month and require 1,000 Patients. Different from

Concierge Medicine, the typical DPC fee nationally according to *The DPC Journal* (www.DirectPrimaryCare.com) for a DPC membership is between $50-$100.00 per month.

Due to the complexity and overhead expenses associated with Hybrid Concierge Medicine practices, the DPC business model has been, as of late (2012-2014), an enticing alternative for a number of doctors looking to discontinue local insurer relationships and Medicare billing. On the horizon in the next two years the Editors at *Concierge Medicine Today* and its sister publication, *The DPC Journal*, predict that more consultants will be helping Hybrid Concierge Medicine physicians move their practices into a DPC medical model.

"What is the thing that Patients appreciate the most about my practice? Accessibility. If they need me, they can reach me. In fact, I just answered a question for a Patient right before I wrote this sentence. One person had a child with flu-like symptoms on New Year's day and was contemplating taking them to the ER. I told them to meet me at the office and I ran a flu test and took a quick look at them. No big deal; it took me about 10 minutes and I saved an ER visit. This kind of thing happens with regularity (not usually after hours, thankfully), and having an office that at most has one Patient present, it is easy to handle them quickly and efficiently. My only challenge thus far has been to convince people to call me before they go to the ER or urgent care. Many of them still imagine their phone calls or secure messages are "bothering me," despite my reassurance that this is exactly why I charge a monthly fee."

~Rob Lamberts, MD, DPC Physician from Augusta, GA

Technology

The Future Of Primary Care Is In Technology, Accessibility And Price Transparency.

More health technology companies are beginning to provide various kinds of solutions accessibility to doctors. ZocDoc enables online appointment booking and check-ins and Ringadoc supports on-demand video and phone calls with doctors.

One Medical Group, a San Francisco-based medical practice aiming to use technology to deliver concierge-style medicine has raised $30 million in a round led by Google Ventures. Startups offer all sorts of digital health products and services but One Medical Group is using health technology to power an entire health care practice. Recently, the company said it had raised $30 million in a Series F round that brings its total amount raised to $77 million. Google Ventures led the round and previous investors, Benchmark Capital, DAG Ventures, Oak Investment Partners and Maverick Capital, also participated.

Founded in 2005 by MD-turned-MBA, Dr. Tom Lee, One Medical Group aims to bring "concierge"-style medicine to the masses. In addition to more personalized care and same-day visits, Patients can book appointments, renew prescriptions, check lab results and see their medical records online, as well as exchange email with their doctors. "We are trying to make health care work and we think we can do that by building a stronger system... and using technology that lets doctors interact thoughtfully with Patients to manage their health," said Lee.

Dr. Samir Qamar, MedLion's founder and CEO, explains, "As primary care physicians look for ways to enjoy private practice again, DPC (DPC) keeps coming up. DPC allows employers and consumers to enjoy high quality primary care at a fraction of the cost of insurance-based models, with a strong focus on customer service and preventive medicine. For this reason, MedLion is growing around the country also. With practices being prepared and/or operational in several cities.

With the industry's inclusion in the Affordable Care Act (ACA), DPC has already shown to be a strong solution for small- and medium-size businesses, as well as individuals who have been frozen out of the healthcare market by current pricing trends. In addition, the MedLion program benefits companies by lowering worker's compensation premiums.

"Our approach to primary medical care and strong, cost-controlling application of occupational and worker's compensation is a dramatic step for companies. When employers enroll their employees in our MedLion program we can substantially drive down their year-end workman's comp costs," says Dr. Marcus Williams, who joined MedLion inside their first Pennsylvania DPC practice.

Some folks in the health care field are opposed to franchising any branch of medical care. However, we have an era coming with more innovation in health care delivery in our country than we have had in a generation. The way health care is delivered will radically change and the focus will be on you, the customer.'

What About The Impact Of Retail Medicine, Convenient Care Clinics, and the Like In Our Local Neighborhoods?

Driven by both consumer demand and the prospect of new business and professional opportunities, "convenient care"—the collective term for urgent care centers and retail clinics— is a major development in the delivery of ambulatory care and a support tool of primary care. At the time this book was being published, a 2015 report from The United Hospital Fund in New York was published which stated that 'Urgent care centers and retail clinics insert an interesting twist in an emerging story. They represent, potentially, a step back from the ideal of a team of providers working together to coordinate care, focus on wellness and prevention, and better manage quality, continuity, and costs. As such, it is vital that we understand their implications, and consider how policymakers, payers, and other providers might best respond.

In looking to the literature on convenient care nationally, and assessing its status, The UHF sought to connect the dots between this recent development and the restructuring, throughout the health care system, of how care is delivered, paid for, and coordinated. They found not only possible points of conflict but, as important, ways that convenient care might support primary care.

Retail medicine and price transparency are quite possibly the future of affordable health care in the U.S. Like most large pharmacies, the creators of 'Retail Medicine' understood years ago the need for affordable, convenient and price-driven access to healthcare.

Until retail and Concierge Medicine came along, people would blindly walk into a doctor's office or hospital and not know (or in many cases, care) about how much things cost. We do not purchase our homes, our vehicles or other services in this way. It is time we stop using our health insurance card as a form of credit.

A significant number of modern medical centers and physicians across the country are now starting to show their prices to their Patients before they sit down for a visit. Dermatology offices and DPC clinics are a good example. Until recently, hospitals, primary care and other health care specialties were one of the only segments in the U.S. that rarely listed how much their fees were for their time, services and products.

"Maybe we should be examining why our Patients would rather go to a retail clinic than see us (their primary care doctors)," says Dr. Robert Nelson. "Here are just a few of the comments I hear from urgent care (UC) Patients as to why they come to the retail healthcare centers instead of their primary care physician: my physician couldn't get me in; my physician does not do stitches anymore; my physician does not do x-rays in office; my physician does not take walk-in Patients; my physician usually refers me to specialist for everything anyway; and my physician won't return my calls."

As the healthcare system is beginning to cope with an influx of 30 million Americans who will have health coverage as a result of the Affordable Care Act, a surging market of retail clinics is poised to take on a wider role to relieve the bottleneck. According to a recent article by Bill Malone in the AACC, he writes *'Retail clinics are also adding new tests that go far beyond caring for scraped knees and scratchy throats. The growing list of tests includes lipid panels, HbA1c, microalbumin, HIV, fecal occult blood, influenza A and B, and even screening for methicillin-resistant Staphylococcus aureus. Clinics offer many of these tests as part of adult and child physicals, and more recently, Medicare wellness visits, and more.'*

The article also notes that *the expected influx of newly insured Patients under the Affordable Care Act provides both opportunity and uncertainty for the retail clinic model, according to the lead author of the study, Ateev Mehrotra, MD.*

"If more people are seeking primary care, and there is no dramatic increase in the number of primary care physicians, we could face a situation of increased demand and worsening access. Without an alternative, more Patients may go to a retail clinic," he said. "The flipside is that a significant segment of Patients who go to a retail clinic do not have a primary care physician. If under healthcare reform more people gain access to primary care physicians, it is still possible they could choose the physician's office over the retail clinic." Mehrotra is a policy analyst at the RAND Corporation and an associate professor of medicine at the University of Pittsburgh School of Medicine.

According to Dr. Jeffrey Cain, family physicians have responded to the demand for greater flexibility by expanding access to appointments. "Family doctors have responded so that about 75 percent of their offices have open-access, same-day appointments and about half have evening or weekend office hours," he said. Results from an AAFP physician survey also found that about 31% of respondents offered weekend appointments. Both the AMA and AAFP are urging insurers not to give Patients an incentive to use retail clinics, warning of the potential for duplicative tests and treatments, higher costs, and lower quality.

As retail clinics have grown in number and ventured into the sphere of chronic disease management, they have also met with stern criticism from some physician groups, such as the American Medical Association (AMA) and the American Academy of Family Physicians (AAFP). AAFP has been vocal in opposing any expansion of the scope of service in retail clinics that approaches managing chronic conditions. It believes that high quality and coordinated care depend on relationships with primary care physicians—a relationship with which retail clinics interfere.

"AAFP believes that the best healthcare comes from a Patient-centered medical home, where you have a strong primary care focus with comprehensive, coordinated, and continuing care," said Dr. Cain. "When retail clinics start talking about managing chronic disease or performing well adult exams, that is further fragmenting an already fragmented health system. We believe Patients will have better care and better quality if they find that care within an ongoing relationship to a primary care physician who knows that person."

The National Landscape

According to data analyzed from nearly 1,000 currently operating concierge practices in the U.S. between 2011 and 2013, we have determined the national average annual fee for concierge medical services is between $1,400-$1,800 per Patient per year. Large networks of Concierge Medicine and DPC doctors have claimed a significant portion of the Concierge Doctor market share and thus help to keep prices from inflating too high in major metropolitan markets. Due to competition, we have found that some independent Concierge Doctors, those not affiliated with the larger franchise consulting companies, who are not part of a large group may charge higher rates, $2,500 and up.

According to industry physicians and business leaders currently operating in this market space, this price difference is primarily due to the fact that franchise Concierge Medicine practices are better supported during the initial launch period and do a better job of educating Patients about what services will be included for the fee. Therefore, more Patients sign-up by start-up. Meanwhile, independent physicians who do it themselves, are, at times, struggling to acquire the necessary amount of Patients to support operational activities, thus, many are charging more per month for their services because they have less Patients and less start-up support to help them with strategic planning, messaging and growth.

Some programs cost as little as $10 per month for children. Patients typically receive unlimited access to the doctor at their home, work or the doctor's office along with unlimited technology visits, such as cell phone, web cam, email and texting. Furthermore, many concierge and DPC doctors offer access to wholesale pricing on prescriptions, lab tests, imaging services and medical supplies for pennies on the dollar. One example recently seen was by a primary care physician in Atlanta, GA who has negotiated a CAT Scan through a local healthcare facility for his Patients for only $150.

"Do not be afraid to try something new. If we do not try to do things differently, primary care will continue to languish and we will have a harder and harder time attracting people into the field and ensuring that primary care survives for us, our children, and our grandchildren. You do not have to do it all at once, though – a lot of practices are trying to develop a hybrid model, gradually moving more and more of their Patients to the DPC model. It is challenging to do this if you are caring for large numbers of Patients, but practices are finding ways to do it." -Dr. Erika Bliss of Qliance.

The Pricing Conundrum: Will Fees Be Going Up Or Down? And Where?

Currently, fees are actually going down among independent, non-franchised concierge physicians, while fees are going up inside those doctors' offices operating within a franchised concierge medical support system.

So, why is this the case if fees among non-franchised, independent Concierge Doctors are higher? Well, since the November 2012 election and the Affordable Care Act (ACA) moving into full implementation, more Patients are seeking to lock-in a relationship and membership at a medical practice that offers transparent pricing and a plethora of services. The number of Patients who are seeking concierge medical care is far greater than the actual number of primary care and family practice doctors available to serve them.

Despite what is heard from the media about the increase in concierge and private-pay physicians growing across America, there are simply not enough of these [Concierge Medicine, direct care or membership medicine-style] physicians currently operating to meet the current demand. Interest in *Concierge Medicine Today*'s national directory, exclusively for Concierge Medicine and DPC physicians in the U.S. who are accepting new Patients has increased tremendously since the 2012 election. But, unfortunately, even if you include all of the doctors touting themselves as retainer-based or concierge medical practices — at the end of the day, the marketplace is still falling short.

There are currently four states that have a huge lead in the number of active concierge or private-pay physicians in practice and consumers seeking their care. Florida, California, Pennsylvania and Virginia each have a significant number of people [most over age 50] seeking out Concierge Doctors and there is, fortunately, a sizeable number of concierge physicians to serve them. It is in these areas where we are seeing franchise Concierge Medicine fees increase and independent Concierge Doctor fees decrease due to competition, Patient demand for transparency and the effect of the ACA in the national marketplace.

Interviews with various physicians and industry sources indicate that the average Patient or consumer of Concierge Medicine and DPC services can withstand a small annual premium increase of about $25 to $160 per year. However, the problem with raising prices for Concierge Medicine Patients, especially in private, DPC medicine and small medical clinics is that it causes Patients to reassess how much value this care brings to their life. They also have other factors to consider such as their financial commitments, their current quality of life, recent good or bad experiences with the doctors' staff, traffic, and interruptions and how often do they actually utilize services on an annual basis.

"I do not foresee any rate increases for 2015," says Dr. Rob Nelson of Cumming, GA to one of his Patients. "I do not expect an increase in my costs for Lab or X-ray, so that component probably won't be an issue. Unless my medical supply costs go up significantly, I do not foresee any price increases for 2015. For your peace of mind, I will guarantee that you can renew with no more than 5% increase."

We receive inquiries every day from people looking to join a Concierge Medicine practice. We also regularly receives inquiries from doctors who are looking at how much they are charging for services. They are attempting to determine how they can balance those fees and still charge what their Patients will pay without appearing to price-gouge their Patients.

States with Doctors Considering Starting A Concierge Medicine Medical Practice

Merritt Hawkins released similar data from their survey among physicians considering opening a concierge medical practice stating the following:

- Texas: 10.6 percent
- Florida: 9.1 percent
- New York: 8 percent
- California: 6.7 percent
- North Carolina: 5.6 percent
- Illinois: 5.3 percent
- Washington State: 4.8 percent
- Pennsylvania: 4.5 percent

Increasing the Number of Concierge Physicians Across The U.S.

While the number of physicians entering concierge medical practices needs to increase, more transparent pricing among doctors is also needed. Unfortunately, our nation's new health care reform law does little in this respect.

Our opinion is that there are approximately 12,000+ physicians nationwide operating in a Concierge Medicine, DPC or retainer-based practice. There are however, three ways we see that will instantly increase the number of physicians stated above.

First, understand that the terminology being used in the Concierge Medicine or DPC marketplace describes many types of business models where doctors have some form of non-insurance or direct financial relationship with their Patients. While all Concierge Medicine practices share similarities, they may vary widely in their structure, payment requirements, and form of operation. But at the end of the day, price transparency, access, affordable rates and the personal level of service provided to each Patient is what they all have in common.

Second, understand that the term Concierge Medicine and DPC describes more specialties than just primary care, internal medicine and family medicine. Some dermatology, pediatric, psychiatry, urology, cardiology and even dental practitioners are now providing forms of concierge medical care.

Third, education. Most people understand that Concierge Medicine and DPC has had somewhat of a "brand/identity" issue. Concierge Medicine has been seen as medical care for the rich, albeit, that impression has changed dramatically in the past 48 months throughout the media. DPC on the other hand has not gotten enough discussion in the local, regional or national media. These delivery models have been referred to as: membership medicine; boutique medicine; retainer-based medicine; concierge health care; cash only practice; direct care; DPC, personalized healthcare, direct practice medicine and, most recently, contract carrying healthcare. At its inception, it appeared to be costly, elitist and controversial, therefore, many people associated a "rich man's" stigma to it. However, the consumer, the physician community and even some legislators are realizing that this form of healthcare delivery, when free-market driven, is saving money and providing "better care," according to MDVIP hospitalization studies reported over the past two years.

What's interesting about DPC as of late (Fall 2014), is that the medias objections to DPC are the same as that of Concierge Medicine from just five years ago. Patient abandonment, smaller panel sizes and membership fees.

Update! New Study Conducted by Optum and MDVIP Finds Personalized Preventive Care Significantly Reduces Healthcare Expenditures Among Medicare Advantage Beneficiaries. Read More ...
http://conciergemedicinenews.wordpress.com/2014/09/09/mdvip-study-new-study-conducted-by-optum-and-mdvip-finds-personalized-preventive-care-significantly-reduces-healthcare-expenditures-among-medicare-advantage-beneficiaries/

The recent Merritt Hawkins Study released in January 2013 tells us that growth in the physician marketplace for doctors expecting to transition into concierge or private-pay medicine is at less than seven percent. While this will keep some consultants busy for the next couple of years, the marketplace consumer is a long way from seeing a Concierge Doctor in every neighborhood. Regardless of how you describe it or the term you associate with Concierge Medicine, the public's perception of these healthcare delivery models is changing for the better. Patient retention among concierge medical physicians is 7 to 9 years, two years longer than traditional, insurance-based primary care practices. We expect this number to increase as time passes and more data becomes available. When a physician is free to create pricing structures that meet their local demographic demands without the intrusion from insurance and avoid providing "hamster healthcare," which only allows doctors to spend 6 to 9 minutes with their Patients, you make a happier Patient, healthier family and less frustrated and fatigued doctor who is able to care for their Patients more thoroughly and comprehensively.

Average Monthly Cost Of A Concierge Doctor In U.S.
The Concierge Medicine Research Collective, ConciergeMedicineToday.com

- Less than $50/mo. – Eleven percent (11%) of surveyed concierge medical practices.
- $51-$100/mo. – Nearly fourteen percent (14%) of surveyed concierge medical practices.
- $101-$135/mo. – Nearly thirty-one percent (31%) of surveyed concierge medical practices.
- $135-$180/mo. – Less than nine percent (<9%) of surveyed concierge medical practices.
- $181-$225/mo. – Less than one percent (<1%) of surveyed concierge medical practices.
- $226+/mo. – Nearly thirty-five percent (34%) of surveyed concierge medical practices.

However, high-deductible health care plans accompanied by a Concierge Medicine doctor or DPC monthly membership at a local clinic are no longer a novelty—they are becoming mainstream.

If more people are exposed to the cost value of concierge medical care, it will make a big difference in what they spend. A recent story in a widely popular national newspaper supports this belief. The paper reports that the State of Indiana has a high-deductible plan and another that is a traditional HMO. People in the high-deductible plan spend thousands less than those in the HMO.

'The average expense in 2009 for Patients in one of these [high-deductible] plans was $6,393,' the paper writes, 'compared with $8,570 for Patients enrolled in a more traditional health maintenance organization plan.'

According to the industry trade group America's Health Insurance Plans, the number of people with these kind of high-deductible plans reached more than 11.4 million in January 2011, up from 10 million in January 2010.

In 2012, a survey from the Kaiser Family Foundation found that about half of all workers in "small" businesses (up to 199 workers) who have health insurance have these plans.

According to the Kaiser Foundation, the average expense in 2012 is $6,050 for an individual and $12,100 for a family. Out-of-pocket costs generally include the deductible, the Patient's share of the cost of seeing a doctor, prescription medicines and/or hospital costs.

Update! An early look at the cost of health insurance in 16 major cities finds that average premiums for the benchmark silver plan – the one upon which federal financial help under the Affordable Care Act to consumers is based – will decrease slightly in 2015. The new study from the Kaiser Family Foundation analyzes premiums in the largest cities in 15 states and the District of Columbia where information from rate filings is available.

The recent analysis finds that in nearly all of the 16 areas studied, a single 40-year-old with income of $30,000 a year would pay 0.8 percent less in premiums in 2015 than in 2014 to enroll in the second-lowest-cost silver plan, after taking tax credits into account.

For bronze-level plans, which cover about 60 percent of enrollees' health expenses on average, the analysis finds that the premium for the lowest-cost bronze option across the marketplaces is increasing an average of 3.3 percent in 2015. Here again changes vary across areas, from a decline of 15.7 percent in the premium (to $196 per month) for the lowest-cost bronze plan available in Hartford, Conn., to a premium increase of 13.3 percent (to $165 per month) for such a plan in Baltimore. Bronze plans are the least expensive option someone can choose to satisfy the ACA's requirement to have coverage.

Source: http://kff.org/health-reform/press-release/premiums-set-to-decline-slightly-for-benchmark-aca-marketplace-insurance-plans-in-2015/

Here's the upshot: When you combine high-deductible health plan policies with a concierge medical program, you empower people and families to make better decisions about their health care, they in turn receive more comprehensive medical care and then the savings happen and stronger relationships occur between the physician and their Patients. Doctors can feel good about the care and time dedicated to helping their patients. One concierge physician said it best when she said that her Patients can say *'I no longer have a doctor who needs to look at my chart to know my name.'*

"In selecting only a small population of clients and providing dedicated counseling sessions, sometimes as often as weekly, allows clients to actively participate in their care plan and to move goals forward at a real-time pace. This enables all of us to realize that healthcare can be a positive experience."

~Dr. Carrie Bordinko, Concierge Physician, Paradise Valley, AZ

"There was a time when patients valued their family doctor, trusted our opinion and called us after hours to help decide if symptoms needed urgent attention or could wait," says Dr. Ellie Campbell of Campbell Family Medicine in Cumming, GA in an interview with Concierge Medicine Today. "Our phone trees, answering services, and after hours call-sharing doctors make it unlikely that any given patient will actually speak to their own doctor. So they don't bother, and they seek care wherever it is most convenient."

BOOM TOWNS

BEST CITIES in AMERICA FINDING SUCCESS IN DIRECT PRIMARY CARE 2014
Based On Patient Searches & CONSUMER DEMAND

By The Direct Primary Care Journal, 2013-2014 | All Content Copyright © 2014. .

Historically, niche industries developed in certain cities due to access to raw materials (think Pittsburgh and Steel), distribution (any major port city), climate (Hollywood sunshine and movies), educational institutions (Stanford and tech), or cheap labor (Alabama and cars).* Today, some of those same forces are in place, but several new ones have risen up to influence healthcare spending. Where and why certain healthcare delivery models and specialized medical practices have clustered -- thrived -- and today, provide political security are now known. Revolutionary new laws, such as the legislation of retainer based practices in Michigan and Louisiana and Washington, are giving rise to the development of new healthcare delivery models -- i.e. Direct Primary Care. The result is a diverse collection of cities with the increasing consumer demand to support such free market medicine businesses to match. (Sources: The Direct Primary Care Journal, 2015; *Entrepreneur.com, August 2014)

DPC BOOM TOWNS = Orange

CONCIERGE MEDICINE BOOM TOWNS = Blue

MOST POPULAR CITIES in AMERICA FOR PATIENT/CONSUMERS SEARCHES for DIRECT PRIMARY CARE and CONCIERGE PHYSICIANS in 2014

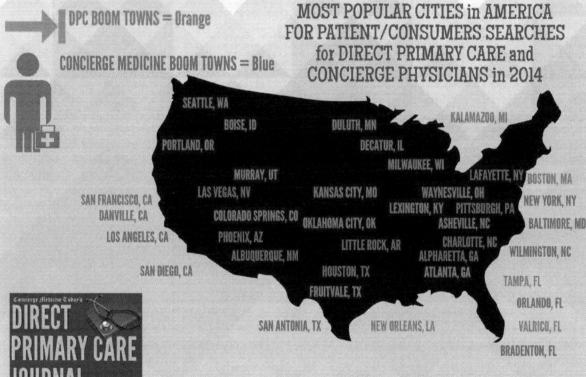

SEATTLE, WA
BOISE, ID
PORTLAND, OR
MURRAY, UT
SAN FRANCISCO, CA
LAS VEGAS, NV
DANVILLE, CA
COLORADO SPRINGS, CO
LOS ANGELES, CA
PHOENIX, AZ
ALBUQUERQUE, NM
SAN DIEGO, CA

DULUTH, MN
DECATUR, IL
MILWAUKEE, WI
KANSAS CITY, MO
OKLAHOMA CITY, OK
LITTLE ROCK, AR
HOUSTON, TX
FRUITVALE, TX
SAN ANTONIA, TX
NEW ORLEANS, LA

KALAMAZOO, MI
LAFAYETTE, NY
WAYNESVILLE, OH
LEXINGTON, KY   PITTSBURGH, PA
ASHEVILLE, NC
CHARLOTTE, NC
ALPHARETTA, GA
ATLANTA, GA

BOSTON, MA
NEW YORK, NY
BALTIMORE, MD
WILMINGTON, NC
TAMPA, FL
ORLANDO, FL
VALRICO, FL
BRADENTON, FL

Concierge Medicine Today's
DIRECT PRIMARY CARE JOURNAL

Cities Identified By The Direct Primary Care Journal, 2013-2014 DOC FINDER SEARCH ENGINE Filtered Over 3,843 Patient Searches | All Content Copyright © 2014. .

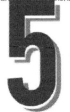

5 MIN GUIDE:

We Asked 750+ DPC and
Concierge Medicine
Doctors What They
Thought ...

WHAT MAKES DPC DIFFERENT FROM CONCIERGE MEDICINE?

INFOGRAPHIC DESIGNED & CREATED By The Direct Primary Care Journal, 2012-2014 and Concierge Medicine Today, 2009-2014
www.DirectPrimaryCare.com | www.ConciergeMedicineToday.com | All Content Copyright © 2014. Concierge Medicine Today, LLC.

Patient Panel Size in DPC Clinics

Generation X is Patient Demographic Using DPC Clinics Most Throughout The U.S. In 2012-2014

64%
of DPC practices said they have less than 400 Patients In The Practice Subscribing to Monthly Memberships.

<$95k/Yr.

The majority of patients that participate in a DPC practice, approximately 59%, earn a combined annual household income of less than $95,000. Gen. X makes up a growing percentage of patients in this industry. The Millennial Generation, is not far behind as a prominent demographic finding DPC popular. Generation X, encompass a population of 44 to 50 million Americans. Now that Generation X is all grown up, they are the latest group of adult children trending towards utilizing DPC nationwide, according to The DPC Journal.

Concierge Medicine Patients: 400+ Patient Subscribers /Yr..

68% of Concierge Medicine practices reported they have more 400+ Patients Under Annual Memberships.

Concierge Medicine Median Income: $175,000 CCH/Yr. (Baby Boomers)

In an Interview with CNN Money (Dec. 2014), Michael Tetreault, Editor-in-Chief of Concierge Medicine Today, says "Overall, (63%) of Concierge Medicine patients skew upper middle class, with typical household earnings between $125,000 and $250,000 a year. They also tend to be Baby Boomers, generally in their 50s to 80s, according to doctors interviewed."

Monthly Fee Less Than $99/mo.

$ 82%
In total, 82% of DPC Memberships Cost Less Than $99/Mo.

Concierge Medicine $$ Range: $101-$225/Mo.

Only 28% of Concierge Medicine Memberships Cost Less Than $100/mo. The majority (57%) cost patient subscribers between $101-$225/mo.

In total, 82% of DPC Memberships Cost Less Than $99/Mo. Breakdown: 68% of DPC practices cost between $25 to $85 a month. And, 45% of DPC Medical Offices average between $51-$85 per month.

DIRECT PRIMARY CARE JOURNAL

DPC vs. Concierge Medicine COMBINED ANNUAL HH INCOME of PATIENT(S)

63% of DPC Patients/Consumers Earn Less Than $100k per year. By The Direct Primary Care Journal, 2013-2014

33% of Concierge Medicine Patients/Consumers Earn Less Than $100k per year. By Concierge Medicine Today, 2009-2014

We Asked 1,300+ DPC and Concierge
Medicine Patients What They Thought ...

WHAT IS DPC?
WHAT IS CONCIERGE MEDICINE?

SOURCE: The Direct Primary Care Journal, (C) 2014. and Concierge Medicine Today, (C) 2014. All Rights Reserved.

"Confusion arises from similarities that exist in both models, such as decreased patient panels, monthly subscriptions, and longer visits. There is added confusion when a DPC physician offers house calls or email access, typical of concierge practices. Confusion is maximized when a physician is by definition practicing direct primary care, yet calls the practice a "concierge practice.""
~Samir Qamar, MD, CEO, MedLion, August 2014

Direct Primary Care Is ...   ?   ## Concierge Medicine Is ...

Cost: Monthly fees at direct practices vary from $25-$85 per month or less. Patients prefer to pay monthly vs. quarterly or annually.

Who: DPC patients typically come from the Generation X and Millennial population and earn a combined annual HH income of less than $100k.

What: DPC is primary and preventative care, urgent care, chronic disease management and wellness support through a monthly care fee patients (or an employer) pay to cover the specific primary care preventative care services.

How: DPC practices are distinguished from other retainer-based care models, such as concierge care, by lower retainer fees, which cover at least a portion of primary care services provided in the DPC practice. No insurance plan is involved, although patients may have separate insurance coverage for more costly medical services.

A DPC health care provider charges a patient a set monthly fee for all primary care services provided in the office, regardless of the number of visits.

Because the insurance "middle man" is removed from the equation, all the overhead associated with claims, coding, claim refiling, write-offs, billing staff, and claims-centric EMR systems disappears.

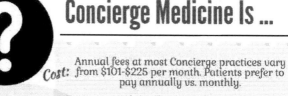

DIRECT PRIMARY CARE JOURNAL

Cost: Annual fees at most Concierge practices vary from $101-$225 per month. Patients prefer to pay annually vs. monthly.

Who: Concierge Medicine patients skew upper middle class, with typical household earnings between $125,000 and $250,000 a year. They also tend to be Baby Boomers, generally in their 50s to 80s, according to doctors interviewed.

What: A greater breadth of primary care services covered by an annual retainer contract fee structure.

How: Many concierge doctors also bill insurance or Medicare for actual medical visits, as the monthly "access fee" is only for "non-covered" services. This results in two subscriptions paid by patients — the concierge medicine fee, and the insurance premium. Importantly, a few concierge practices do not bill insurance for medical visits, as the monthly fees cover both access and primary care visits.

Roughly 12,000 doctors practice concierge medicine with an estimated 1.5 million patients nationwide. Why so few? Tetreault, Editor of The DPC Journal and Concierge Medicine Today, separate trade journals for the industry, chalks it up to a PR problem. "People really don't understand that it's affordable, that it's not just for the rich." And they can be hard to find: In more rural areas like South Dakota or Mississippi, sometimes only a handful of doctors serve an entire state. And while critics question its basic fairness — Are the rich getting healthier while the poor get sicker? — concierge doctors say they can now spend more time helping patients, less time mucking with paperwork, and they point to new studies suggesting it can actually lower the cost of health care.

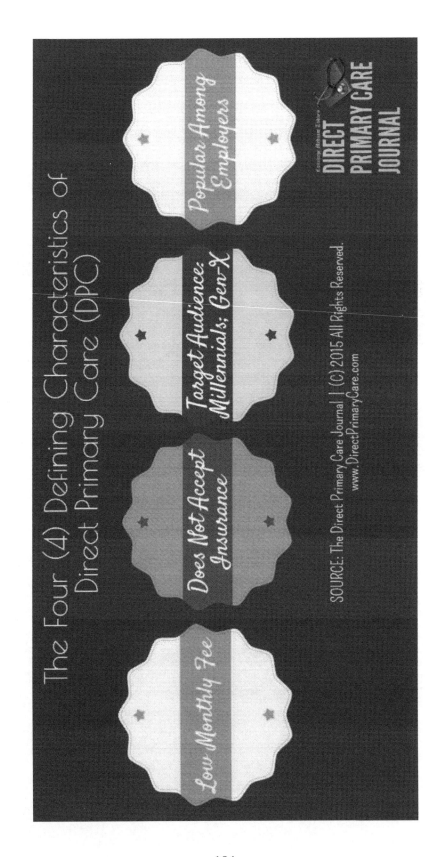

The Four (4) Defining Characteristics of Direct Primary Care (DPC)

Popular Among Employers

Target Audience: Millennials; Gen-X

Does Not Accept Insurance

Low Monthly Fee

DIRECT PRIMARY CARE JOURNAL

ADVICE

By The Direct Primary Care Journal, 2013-2014 and Concierge Medicine Today, 2009-2014 | All Content Copyright © 2014, Concierge Medicine Today, LLC.

FOR DOCTORS

"Don't apologize to your patients for the business changes you're making. This new process will help them. Inform them that this is a positive change and will help you maintain more secure patient-physician communication on a timely basis and offers them a much more affordable payment system with routine and convenient access to their doctor."
~Mike Permenter, Industry Consultant

FOR SPECIALTY DOCTORS

"The anti-aging and medical home delivery model fits well inside a concierge medicine [and direct care] practice. The nutritional component, the wellness solutions, the anti-aging and team-focused health care delivery professionals led by a concierge [or direct care] doctor are providing comprehensive and continuous health care services to patients year after year that they simply can't find elsewhere. This combination is increasing patient retention and patient interest in the concept. The goal here is healthy outcomes for patients followed by increased patient retention outcomes for the physician year after year." ~Michael Tetreault, Editor, CMT, The DPC Journal

FROM A DOCTOR to a DOCTOR

"Slow and steady growth is ideal in this type of practice because it allows you to offer patients a personalized experience," says Joel Bessmer, MD, FACP of Omaha, Nebraska's Members.MD.

FROM A CONSULTANT to a DOCTOR

"Typically, there's a period after start-up when income goes way down as patients decide whether to stay," said Allison McCarthy, a senior consultant in the northeast office of Corporate Health Group, a national consulting firm. "It often takes a good two years to bring the patient level up to where it should be." At that point, physicians do better financially. In the interim, they are likely to struggle, particularly with those large start-up costs, which range from $50,000 to over $300,000.

DIRECT PAY

Can it lower your costs?

The Direct Primary Care Coalition estimates that payer-related costs add up to 40 cents of every healthcare dollar in a practice. Eliminating insurance from primary care, according to the coalition, "makes that 40 cents available for actual healthcare—more time with each patient, more extensive office hours, more on-site services and diagnostics, and more patient-provider support technology."

PRIMARY CARE PRACTICE
INSURANCE-BASED REVENUE

Insurance consumes
more than
40 CENTS
of each dollar

- Insurer Profit
- Insurer claim processing
- Practice claim processing
- PRACTICE PROFIT
- Practice non-claim overhead
- Practice provider labor

100%

80%

60%

40%

20%

0%

Source: Direct Primary Care Coalition

CHALLENGES

By The Direct Primary Care Journal, 2013-2014
and Concierge Medicine Today, 2009-2014 | All Content Copyright © 2014, Concierge Medicine Today, LLC.

Medical Centers

"The challenges of medical center concierge-style programs are very different than those experienced by concierge physicians in private practice. All hospitals/medical centers have special perks and usually enhanced access to specialists for their donors and patrons, often a special number they can call. Most have an informal "private banking" approach where there is no established fee, just an expected level of donation. Despite the proliferation of individual concierge practices and now organized networks, concierge medicine programs INSIDE medical centers are quite unusual — there may be only 20-25 in the entire country." ~ John Kirkpatrick, MD Seattle, WA

Insurance Participation

"Direct Primary Care (DPC) is not insurance, does not strive to replace health insurance, nor is it adversarial to it. On the contrary, many DPC practices are eager to work with insurance carriers to co-create blended plans which integrate DPC with high-deductible insurance and ultimately correct the perverse incentives which are rife in the traditional fee-for-service system." ~Dr. David Z. Tusek, Nextera Healthcare, Colorado

"I don't know of a concierge medicine practice in the country who enjoys the headaches of dealing with the third party payor system, but they do so as a convenience to their members. If you see the revenue collected vs. the cost to collect scenarios you may be surprised." ~By Sonja Horner, Healthcare Business Innovator

Marketing & Target Audience Identification

"Dreams are built early in the morning. Countless interviews over the years from successful doctors in the marketplace tell us they measure their ROI and success on the amount of time they spend building their practice to 'be better' than it was yesterday. In today's healthcare culture, the 55-plus audience hasn't been entirely abandoned, but the advertising aimed at this population segment is simply aimed at maintaining brand loyalty and establishing that the products they love are still good, still function and most likely being improved. Conversely, you can watch any prime-time television show that's targeting the 25-54 demographic, and you will learn what those people think is cool, hip, and where our culture is trending. You will not see advertising aimed at the 55-plus demographic population that's designed to get them to switch brands. The advertising aimed at 25-54 is all about that." ~Michael Tetreault, Editor-In-Chief, Concierge Medicine Today and its healthcare trade journal companion, The Direct Primary Care Journal

Retail Medicine

"Patients value speed and low cost most of all for most minor complaints," notes Dr. Ellie Campbell of Cumming, GA. "Even my patients who pay a membership fee for all of their covered and non-covered services including 24-hour access to my personal email and cell phone number, and whose care for these complaints would be covered without additional cost, still use these [retail medicine style] health providers [i.e. CVS, MinuteClinic, TakeCare Clinic, etc.]. Many patients say, 'I just did not want to bother you on the weekend, and I was near there anyhow.' As long as we live in a world of drive-though windows, ATMs, and garage door openers, patients are going to value and pay for any service that gets them in and out quickly, on their time schedule, with their desired objective. We [Concierge Medicine and Direct-Pay Doctors] need to learn to adapt, as this delivery model of care seems here to stay. Unless we offer on site dispensaries, extended hours, and no appointment needed delivery, we will be deferring more urgent issues to these models. Perhaps then we will have more time to devote to preventing disease and reversing the burden of chronic conditions, if only we can convince third party payors that there is value in that."

Set Realistic Expectations

"The people who can pull this off are often people who already have long-term existing practices," says Internist Garrison Bliss, MD, a movement pioneer, sits on the board of the Direct Primary Care Coalition and is Founder and Chief Medical Officer of Seattle-based Qliance Medical Management, the nation's first direct primary care practice. "You need to have 10-15 years in practice, so you have an established base of patients who trust and like you. It also matters if you have people with chronic illnesses, or who are older, who just don't want to go through the heartbreak and complexity of finding another doctor," he continues. "And it depends on whether you really do provide extraordinary service already. The practices that do great work, have large patient populations, have been around for a long time, and have great reputations can often make this transition without difficulty."

"Business is tough," says Dr. Chris Ewin of 121MD in Fort Worth, TX. "If you are doing something just for the money, you are never going to enjoy it. You will be the hardest boss you have ever had. So, find something you love and pursue it. Follow this advice and you will set yourself up for an enjoyable future in medicine."

The Price Is Wrong.

"The biggest mistake in my opinion is charging too low," says Mike Permenter, industry consultant. "Conversions [into this private-pay marketplace] will eventually be unnecessary as the public becomes more aware of the benefits of these types of memberships. The big challenge is continuing growth after the initial conversion. Customer service, as described by some physicians, is the number one way to grow [this type of] practice. Linking the service to local self-insured employers is a good way to grow but certainly requires expertise with regards to structuring the appropriate benefit, usually a high-deductible plan with an HSA plus a membership."

Good Versus Bad Press
About Concierge Medicine In The Media

■ Good Press   ■ Negative Press   ■ Indifferent

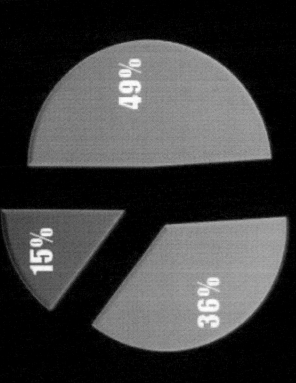

By The Direct Primary Care Journal, 2013-2014
and Concierge Medicine Today, 2009-2014
All Content Copyright © 2014. Concierge Medicine Today, LLC.

"We believe — and this is after years of verifying doctors, talking with actual doctors, talking with business leaders, and talking with physicians who are influencers — that there are slightly less than 4000 physicians who are verifiably, actively practicing concierge medicine or direct primary care across the United States, with probably another 8000 practicing under the radar,"

—Michael Tetreault, Cash-Only Practices: 8 Issues to Consider – Medscape

DPC Finds Foothold In Rural Areas Whereas It Struggles Against Retail Medicine Market Forces In Metro Areas. Concierge Medicine Meanwhile, Does Well In Metropolitan Cities With Adequate Population To Support Its Price Point. It's not impossible, but it's difficult to find a DPC or Concierge Medicine Physician in Rural States Like: Idaho; North Dakota; South Dakota; Louisiana and Mississippi.

—The Direct Primary Care Journal, 2014

"Interviews with various industry sources indicates that the average patient or consumer of concierge medical services market can withstand a small annual premium increase of about $25 to $160 per year," note Concierge Medicine Research Collective Staff. "The problem with raising prices for concierge patients, especially in private, direct-pay medicine and concierge medical clinics is that it causes patients to reassess how much value this care brings to their life, their financial commitment, their current quality of life, past experiences with the doctors' staff, traffic and travel interruptions and how often they actually utilize services on an annual basis."

—Concierge Medicine Research Collective, 2009-2014

Fast Facts

About Direct Primary Care

STRUGGLING STATES

NATIONAL FIGURES 12k

PRICING REFLECTS INFLATION

STARTUP SUCCESS

ENROLLMENT

90% indicated that their practices are doing better financially over one year ago, whereas, only 10% said they were doing worse.

—The Direct Primary Care Journal, 2014

Many new patients will sign up for a monthly membership to a DPC practice in January through March of each year. The DPC Journal reports that August and September are also popular months for membership medicine program enrollment.

—The Direct Primary Care Journal, 2014

FUNDING SOURCES

INSIDE CONCIERGE MEDICINE and DPC CLINICS INCLUDE:

By The Direct Primary Care Journal, 2013-2014 and Concierge Medicine Today, 2009-2014

67% Individual Membership(s) Fund Operations

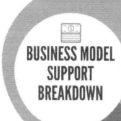

BUSINESS MODEL SUPPORT BREAKDOWN

7% Employer Sponsored Memberships Fund Operations

26% Privately Funded Thru Capital Infusion To Maintain Operations (i.e. Investor Supported, 401k, realestate, etc.)

NOTABLE TRENDS

- Specialty Concierge Medicine Popularity Increasing. Approx. 41% of Identified Concierge Doctors Operate In Specialty Medicine (i.e. Pediatric, Dental, Anti-Aging, Surgery, OBGYN)

- DPC Model Trends Operated Primarily Inside Internal Medicine and Family Medicine Solo Clinics.

- 40% of DPC Doctors Would Not Advise Medical Residents To Enter Into DPC Out of Medical School. Physician Respondents Say 'Requires Knowledge of Payor/Payee issues with the healthcare marketplace.'

- Most Common PPOs Retained After Conversion Are BlueCross and Aetna.

- Technology Innovation Rapidly Expanding In Concierge Medicine and DPC Marketplace. Particularly In EMR, Membership Billing Solutions and Employer Health Tracking.

- Concierge Medicine Seen As A Viable Retirement Option With Average Age of Most Concierge Doctors Age 60+

- DPC Business Model Becoming Increasingly Popular For Physicians Age 45-59

- Significant Salary Drop First 18-Mos.

- 60% of Patients Prefer To Pay Monthly Wheras 35% of Patients Pay Annual Fee. 5% Prefer Quarterly Billing. Note: Many Doctors Give 10-18% Discount off Annual Fee If Annual Fee Paid In Full

INFOGRAPHIC AND SOURCES
By The Direct Primary Care Journal, 2013-2014
and Concierge Medicine Today, 2009-2014

NOTABLE THREATS to MARKETPLACE

- Overpromised/Under Served Patients In Both DPC and Concierge Medicine Threaten Monthly/Annual Renewals.

- Low Awareness of DPC Among Consumer Audience. To date, buyers of health care know little about the DPC model but understand Concierge Medicine.

- Growth of Retail Medicine In Both Metropolitan and Rural Markets. Note: The Price Point of Most Retail Clinics Appeals To DPCs Patient Population Demographic.

- Many Practices Are Selling Out to Larger Health Systems, Eliminating the Concierge Medicine and DPC Option.

INFOGRAPHIC AND SOURCES
By The Direct Primary Care Journal, 2013-2014
and Concierge Medicine Today, 2009-2014

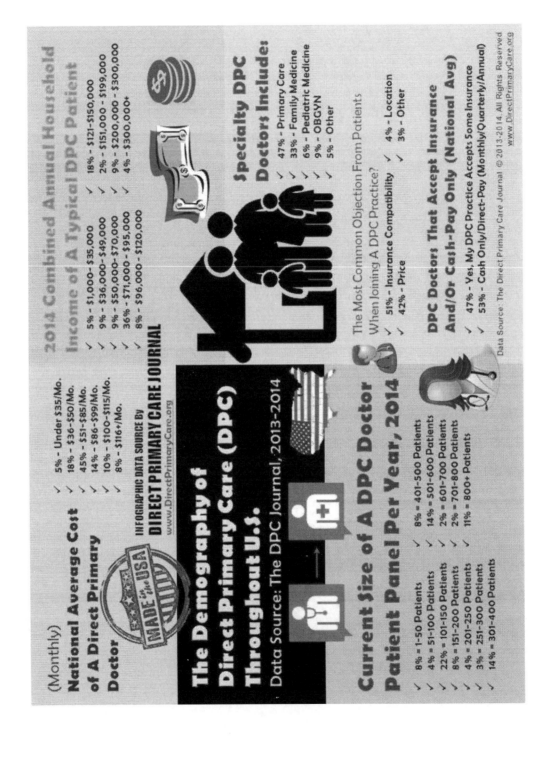

(Monthly)
National Average Cost of A Direct Primary Doctor

- 5% – Under $35/Mo.
- 18% – $36–$50/Mo.
- 45% – $51–$85/Mo.
- 14% – $86–$99/Mo.
- 10% – $100–$115/Mo.
- 8% – $116+/Mo.

INFOGRAPHIC DATA SOURCE By
DIRECT PRIMARY CARE JOURNAL
www.DirectPrimaryCare.org

The Demography of Direct Primary Care (DPC) Throughout U.S.
Data Source: The DPC Journal, 2013–2014

Current Size of A DPC Doctor Patient Panel Per Year, 2014

- 8% = 1–50 Patients
- 4% = 51–100 Patients
- 22% = 101–150 Patients
- 8% = 151–200 Patients
- 4% = 201–250 Patients
- 3% = 251–300 Patients
- 14% = 301–400 Patients
- 8% = 401–500 Patients
- 14% = 501–600 Patients
- 2% = 601–700 Patients
- 2% = 701–800 Patients
- 11% = 800+ Patients

2014 Combined Annual Household Income of A Typical DPC Patient

- 5% – $1,000–$35,000
- 9% – $36,000–$49,000
- 9% – $50,000–$70,000
- 36% – $71,000–$95,000
- 8% – $96,000–$120,000
- 18% – $121–$150,000
- 2% – $151,000–$199,000
- 9% – $200,000–$300,000
- 4% – $300,000+

Specialty DPC Doctors Includes

- 47% – Primary Care
- 33% – Family Medicine
- 6% – Pediatric Medicine
- 9% – OBGYN
- 5% – Other

The Most Common Objection From Patients When Joining A DPC Practice?

- 51% – Insurance Compatibility
- 42% – Price
- 4% – Location
- 3% – Other

DPC Doctors That Accept Insurance And/Or Cash-Pay Only (National Avg)

- 47% – Yes, My DPC Practice Accepts Some Insurance
- 53% – Cash Only/Direct-Pay (Monthly/Quarterly/Annual)

Data Source: The Direct Primary Care Journal © 2013-2014, All Rights Reserved www.DirectPrimaryCare.org

BY DIRECT PRIMARY CARE JOURNAL

www.DirectPrimaryCare.org

Direct Primary Care | HOT ZONES In 2014

Map Looks At Most Popular Urban-Centric Locale Codes of DPC Journal's National Internal Database
of DPC Physician Locations Throughout The U.S. In 2014.

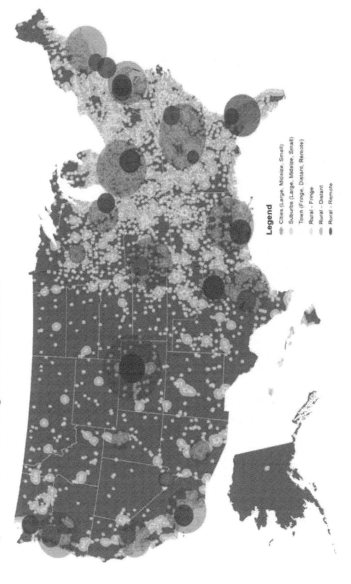

Legend

- Cities (Large, Midsize, Small)
- Suburbs (Large, Midsize, Small)
- Town (Fringe, Distant, Remote)
- Rural - Fringe
- Rural - Distant
- Rural - Remote

Data Sources: 2014, The Direct Primary Care Journal; Urban-Centric Locale Codes.
Developed By The Direct Primary Care Journal; the National Center for Education Statistics (NCES)

BY DIRECT PRIMARY CARE JOURNAL
Direct Primary Care | Search Patterns In 2014

Patient Search Inquires By Urban-Centric Locale Codes For Direct Primary Care Physicians Throughout The U.S.

DPC Journal Physician
Search Inquiries Nationally @
www.DirectPrimaryCare.com
(Jan 10-Dec 10, 2014)

Data Sources: 2014, *The Direct Primary Care Journal*; Urban-Centric Locale Codes.
Developed By www.DirectPrimaryCare.org

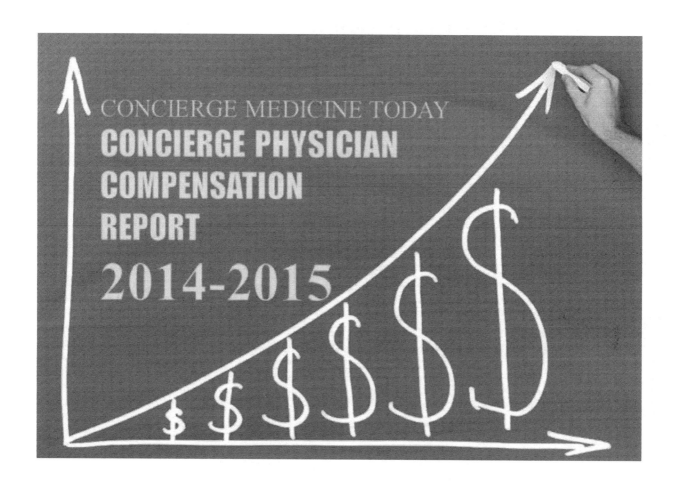

Read Full Analysis at
https://conciergemedicinetoday.org/2015/09/10/concierge-medicine-today-physician-compensation-report-2014-2015/

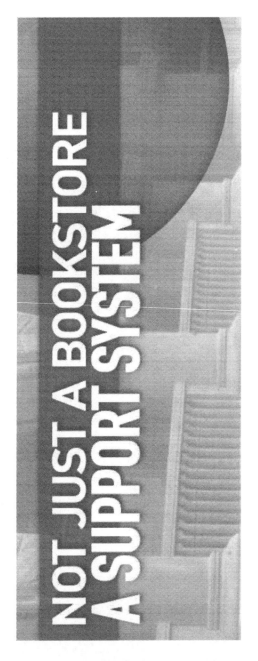

The Docpreneur Institute, Campus Bookstore,
Visit: www.DocpreneurPress.org

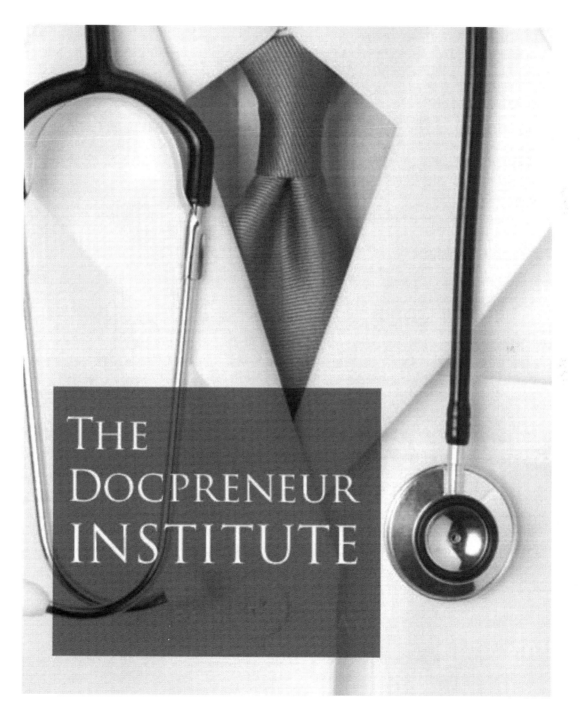

Learn More, Visit: www.TheDocpreneur.org

BIG BRANDS, BIG BACKERS

The vast majority of urgent care clinics are still local mom-and-pops, but investors with deep pockets lust after a Golden Arches-style national brand. Here are the five largest chains:

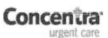	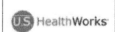	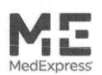		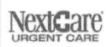
CLINICS **330**	CLINICS **219**	CLINICS **132**	CLINICS **128**	CLINICS **106**
OWNER **HUMANA** (INSURER)	OWNER **DIGNITY HEALTH** (HOSPITAL SYSTEM)	OWNER **SEQUOIA CAPITAL** (VC) **GENERAL ATLANTIC** (PE)	OWNER **INDEPENDENTLY OWNED**	OWNER **ENHANCED EQUITY FUNDS** (PE)

THE DOLLAR MENU

Chest pains mean rushing to the ER, but minor ailments like earaches have a cheaper and friendlier alternative.

	URGENT CARE COST	ER COST	PERCENT SAVINGS
ALLERGIES	$97	$345	72%
ACUTE BRONCHITIS	127	595	79
CHRONIC BRONCHITIS	114	665	83
EARACHE	110	400	73
PHARYNGITIS	94	525	82
PINK EYE	102	370	72
SINUSITIS	112	617	82
STREP THROAT	123	531	77
UPPER RESPIRATORY INFECTION	111	486	77
URINARY TRACT INFECTION	110	665	83

SOURCE: MEDICA HEALTH PLANS.

Cost of Care

A sampling of tests and screenings offered by concierge clinics

Service	Price charged by a lab, hospital or screening facility*	Concierge discount price**
Prostate cancer (PSA) test	$175	$5
Thyroid (TSH levels) test	$94-$125	$10
Routine blood chemistry panel	$46 to $63	$15
Testosterone test	$227	$25
Vitamin D level test	$230	$25
X-Ray	$100	$30-$50
PAP smear	$92	$56
Mammogram	$350	$80
CAT scan	$500 per body part	$150-$470
MRI brain (without contrast)	$600	$380
Colonoscopy	$2,000	$400

* A sampling of what patients pay out-of-pocket, if the test isn't covered by insurance or if the deductible hasn't been met.

** What patients pay directly, without using insurance. Amounts can count toward deductible and out-of-pocket maximums.

Sources: Robert Nelson, MyDoc, Georgia; Tiffany Sizemore-Ruiz, Choice Physicians, Florida; Chris Ewin, 121MD, Texas; Brian Forrest, Access Healthcare, North Carolina; Concierge Medicine Today

Source: http://stream.wsj.com/story/latest-headlines/SS-2-63399/SS-2-378398/

Chapter 4 –
Public Introduction, Part 1.
Learn, Listen & Discover.

If you have made it to this point, you are probably seriously considering this type of medical practice model. However, you need some assurances, some help and to know what to do next. If you have chosen the route of hiring a franchise company or utilizing a conversion consultant, they should tell you what to expect and what happens next. For many, it is assessing your local practice and the feasibility and the likelihood that this will be a success in your practice and geographic area.

The Patient Survey

This survey is conducted to survey your current patient base to determine their satisfaction with your services and receptivity to this concept. Results are obtained in a variety of ways. You can choose to utilize all or just one. If you hire a consultant or a franchise transition company, ask which methods they are going to employ to obtain the data and information you need to make this critical decision. Physicians who have travelled down the road before you advise that this survey should be conducted over a two to three week period and include no less than 250 surveys, phone calls, interviews and/or letters to Patients targeting the ages of 40-50; 51-60; and 60+. In addition, the doctor should choose several Patients with whom he/she has a close relationship and to call those Patients him/herself. This will not only gather data but be a learning experience for the physician in answering questions about this type of practice model and service offering. Physicians and industry experts alike echo the sentiment found by many that says 'the doctor is the best salesperson when it comes to recruiting new Patients to their practice.'

Methods of obtaining survey information may include:

- Telephone surveys conducted by: office staff; the doctor; or a third party brought in by the consultant or hired by the doctor;
- In-office interviews with the Patients before their exam/visit;
- Direct mail letter sent to the selected Patients indicating that the physician is considering a change and would value their input;
- Small group meetings with a presentation from the doctor and a written survey.

There are a number of questions that need to be asked. Although you'd probably like to know the answers to quite a few questions, a simple, short and concise survey is advised by most industry physicians and transition consultants. What you are ultimately wanting to know is which services will your Patients expect, need and/or want if you move forward with a Concierge Medicine, retainer-based or DPC fee practice. You will also find out which services they do not want, which in many cases, is just as important as what they will buy from you later on.

First, it is important that the person conducting the survey (if verbally) be able to articulate what the doctor is considering and why. The emphasis should always be on enhanced patient care and access, not a diatribe on low reimbursements. Although, it can be stated that decreasing reimbursements and administrative difficulties are severely impacting the amount of time the doctor is able to spend treating and helping his/her patients which has become a serious concern for him/her. Having a script to reference is key for whoever will be making these calls – even the doctor.

Questions included in this survey might include:

- Is 24/7 cell phone access to your doctor important?
- On a scale of 1-10, how important are house calls to you?
- Would you like faster appointments with your doctor?
- Would you like to have cell phone and email access to your doctor?
- Would you like online appointment scheduling?
- What services would you want to be included in this new practice design?
- Is specialist coordination and hospital visitation important to you, when necessary?
- What forms of technology would you like to see added to your doctor's practice?
- Is free Wi-Fi in the office important to you?
- If your physician were to switch to a Concierge Medicine, retainer-based or DPC membership model, would you join?
- How much would you be willing to pay for this enhanced access to your doctor?

CASE EXAMPLE: Lessons Learned From A Successful Concierge Medicine and DPC Doctors.

Dr. Jennifer Chilek from Montgomery, TX shares her experience following the transition of her practice. She writes to us (*Concierge Medicine Today*):

"The ability to contact me directly has deepened my relationship with my Patients. They are more apt to confide in me and divulge information that ends up being important to their overall health and wellness. They contact me sooner, rather than later, which seems to improve outcomes. In addition, they are reassured that I am aware of their issue without the overutilization of office visits, minimizing their worry and improving convenience since this is usually via text, email, or our online Patient portal.

Minimizing staff and keeping consistency among contact people has improved our workflow and improved job satisfaction among staff. They feel that Patients or tasks get "lost through the cracks" less often, and they like being able to complete the full circle of an inquiry and pride themselves in Patient satisfaction. I have found that more satisfied Patients means more satisfied staff. Staff burnout from frustrated Patients with billing questions, office communication issues, and problems with referrals and prescriptions has almost disappeared. Our team is getting stronger each month, and I realize this is due to a solid Patient panel that we get to know really well.

I finally have the time to call specialists again! I enjoy being able to interact with them more, follow up on consults, and also contact them for ongoing questions regarding Patient care. I have learned to block off about an hour per day in order to coordinate care with them. In addition, I find myself spending an hour or two on research topics during the day instead of on family time during evenings and weekends."

Do: Start small.

"You can always increase your panel size, but start with a smaller number of Patients in order to ensure you can deliver on promises and expectations. Take a year to grow into the new model to solidify staff and processes. I was surprised at staffing changes that needed to occur after we got the ball rolling with the new practice. Those changes would have been more difficult with a "full" model. However, in the past 6 months, I hired a NP part time. This has given me a lot more flexibility with my schedule and ability to do house and office calls. I plan on expanding our Patient base and "advertising" us as a team. Once you have an established relationship with Patients, they are ok with seeing your partner, as long as they know you are still directly involved.

Currently, we have 350 member Patients. My initial goal was 500, but after realizing the improved quality of life at this level, I am reconsidering my goal. I realize now how much time I was missing with my family and events as they grow up, and time lost with my parents and siblings across the country.

One of the most difficult things I have found is dealing with the feeling of guilt. There are a few reasons guilt comes on strong. First, is the feeling of abandonment. Reducing from 3500 Patients to 350 is drastic. In our smaller town, there aren't many doctors to absorb the Patients. Many PCPs have left the area in the past 9 years since I started my practice, including one from our office. One way I dealt with this guilt is knowing that I had a decision to make-- it was draining me to work the way I did. I could take a business job, have a normal lifestyle, make plenty of money and see NO Patients, or I could change my office and still see 300-500 Patients and take home a modest paycheck. For me, knowing I was ready to quit made this guilt easier to deal with.

The tougher guilt I am having a harder time overcoming is my time "off." As doctors, we are trained early on to work 100 hours per week, non-stop, and 24/7 in and out of the hospital. There is no stopping. We preach to take time for yourself, take care of yourself, etc., but we do not actually get trained to follow that advice. If I am done with paperwork and seeing Patients by 3 pm, I shouldn't feel guilty about leaving the office to go work out, but I do! There is this ingrained sense that your Patients expect you to be there from 8-5 every day, when in reality, they are happy to have you there for them at both of your convenience. My current Patients also understand more than I realized and they are happy for me to take the time with my children, and to stay healthy.

The best way I was able to get the correct information to my Patients about the transition was through small group meetings. We met after hours in my lobby with about 10-15 Patients at a time. They signed up in advance. This gave me an opportunity to explain why I was making the change. Patients wanted to hear it from me, not employees or the concierge company.

Try to keep as much in-house as possible. This related directly to minimizing the number of people your Patients have to talk to. Having to call a call center for one thing, but the office for another is problematic and inconvenient for the staff and the Patient when there is a question.

I was flabbergasted when the first quarterly payment was due from Patients. It was not even time to send the invoice out yet (for those not on automatic credit card payments) and we had Patients calling up asking to pay their membership fee. Six months prior it was like pulling teeth for copays! It is a nice feeling when you know your Patients appreciate you enough to try to pay their bill ahead of time."

Staffing:

"Currently I have our membership coordinator, medical assistant, part time front desk, and part time nurse practitioner. We are changing to a full time PA and eliminating the part time front desk. The full time MA can handle all incoming calls and the PA helps check-in Patients, see Patients when I am not there, and follows up on messages, etc. The membership coordinator is also my "executive secretary" for anything I need, which helps tremendously. Staffing is $200,000 per year. My office overhead is about $5000 per month. I share an office with a full-time traditional doc.

Patients love that I email them every 1-2 weeks. It comes from my personal email account and I keep them up to date on office issues, when I may be out, seasonal information, and I usually add in one or two educational bits. They also love to hear about my kids and what we are up to.

My best friend since third grade was recently diagnosed with breast cancer during her current pregnancy. I had planned our yearly trip to Minnesota to see my family, but found out she was having major surgery the week prior. I flew up from Texas a week early in order to be with her and ended up being away for two weeks. Last year, that would not have been possible. The Patient burden and the lack of income would have been detrimental, but with this model I had no financial problems, and my Patients were happy for me to be able to go. I let them know via email that I was leaving early unexpectedly. They wanted updates on how she was doing. They truly cared. I think I got so callused from the usual brunt of Patient "complaints" and office issues because we were all so stressed that I came to assume the Patients only cared about themselves. I see that mentality across the office with my partner and now I can recognize it. Being pulled in every direction all day every day 100 miles per hour puts everyone on edge and you end up feeling like no one cares how hard you are trying to work for them.

I have to admit, there are a few Patients that I wished would not stay with me. You know, the names you see on the schedule and think "Oh no, I do not have time for this." However, I think those are my most gratifying Patients now. I realize I felt that way before because I never had enough time for them and I was always feeling rushed, but now that I do, their problems do not seem so problematic.

The schedule was interesting in that the first few months after changing, I still saw 8-12 Patients per day. Patients still came in for everything, since they were trained for that all along. 18 months later I had a whopping seven Patients on a Monday after I was out for two weeks. Usually I have 1-5 Patients, occasionally none. I take care of several messages throughout the day, all issues easily handled by phone. I try to see them all before 3 pm and then spend time with my family when they get home from school. I haven't had a call after 7 pm in many months. Once Patients realize you are there for them 24/7, they become less "needy" and much more respectful of your time. On every email I send to them, I encourage them to call my cell if they need anything at any time. I know there are no barriers from the Patients to me. I think a lot of doctors are scared of that, the possible overload of Patient demands, but I have found it exactly opposite."

"An in-depth analysis of our financials revealed we needed to continue operating under the fee-for-service model for the insured Patients, and then introduce the DPC option alongside. We did not want to undermine our existing Patient relationships by declining traditional insurance, but we also wanted a tangible option for Patients who were uninsured or under-insured and forced to seek alternatives due to rising healthcare costs."

- Dr. Clint Flanagan and Dr. David Tusek of Firestone, CO

The Feasibility Analysis.

By now you have probably discovered and learned quite a bit about whether or not your Patients [and staff] are receptive to your vision. You also should have answers to many of the questions you have about exploring the possibility of transitioning to a Concierge Medicine or DPC program in your practice. Dependent upon whether you took it upon yourself to develop a Patient survey or you have chosen to use a consultant to help you discover the answers to your questions, there are a few basic areas that you must be cognizant of prior to reaching the point of, what many doctors call, the point of no return. The questions you should analyze includes (but is not limited to):

- Do you have the right demeanor for this type of business?
- Does this business model and decision excite you, your staff and your spouse?
- Are your Patients receptive to the concept?
- Have you chosen a business model right for your area?
- How many Patients (%-age) will follow you into your new model (estimate low)?
- What is the Service Offering You Will Provide?
- Have you received and become comfortable with one year, two year and 3 year financial forecasting statement(s)?
- Is there a Patient base and a market of sufficient size to make the concept viable?
- Do the capital requirements to start, based on estimates of sales and expenses, make sense?
- Can an appropriate start-up team be put together to execute the concept? This may include: Legal; Insurer Contract Review; Accounting; Billing; HIPAA Compliance; Medicare Compliance; I.T.; Continuation of Care (for those not staying with your practice) and more.
- Have you identified and put together the Strengths, Weaknesses, Opportunities and Threats Analysis (SWOT Analysis) of Current Local Landscape?
- Do you have your Marketing and Communication Message Design?
- Do you have your transition strategy mapped out?

There are a number of other questions that consultants and lawyers will add to this list. We do not presume to have all of them listed here. What is important is the data accumulated and the answers you discover.

One physician in Mission Viejo, California, Dr. Marcela Dominguez started a concierge component in her family medical practice and received data from approximately 1,200 Patients. Her Patient surveys found that roughly 300 would join a Concierge Medicine practice of program. "These were Patients who gave a definite 'yes.' Maybe's did not count. Based on those numbers, we thought my practice had a good chance of succeeding."

Many physicians believe that since most of their Patients have been treated and cared for for years, possibly decades that they will want to spend more time with you and enroll in your new membership Concierge Medicine or DPC program or practice. Regardless of whether you still accept insurance or not, that most likely will not be true. Helen Hadley, Founder and CEO of VantagePoint Healthcare Advisors in Hamden, CT. says "holding on to even one half of your current Patients would be wonderful, but probably not realistic." She notes that converting even 10% of a 3,000 Patient database panel is doing very well. "We like to set up our doctors to make $300,000 a year, but it does not happen right away."

Analyze Patient Demographics: Did you know that female medical doctors' offices fill up more quickly than their male counterparts? Did you know that the average age range for Patients inside a primary care or family medical office is usually within 10-years older or younger than the doctor themselves? These questions along with some local geography and demographic data should be analyzed and assessed. Information on annual Patient income; how many Patients out of your entire Patient data base have visited your practice in the past two years, etc. should be reviewed and considered when making projections.

Develop a Service Offering: The menu and fees you charge will be largely dependent upon your Patients' needs as well as their willingness and ability to pay for a higher level of access and care at your practice.

"It is about believability. Would it work for me? Could it work for me?" says Richard Doughty, CEO of Cypress Concierge Medicine. "In places where physicians have taken an early leap of faith [and started a concierge medical practice], they have been satisfied. As a result, physicians now have many examples of colleagues experiencing the benefits of Concierge Medicine for themselves and their Patients. We see momentum continuing to build."

The key, whether you choose to use a franchise or do-it-yourself, is to go into this private-pay medical marketplace passionate about helping Patients. Even if one type of business model is considered more low risk, remember that businesses close every day. Doctors tell us every day in their editorials and opinion articles that "... *you are going to put a lot of time and money into this endeavor over the next several months, so you need to make sure it is something that you care about.*"

Many doctors start up a Concierge Medicine practice or pursue a career in DPC medicine for a multitude of reasons including: spending more time with Patients; a yearning to use their medical expertise more effectively; a more satisfying lifestyle; and more. Some doctors enter this field of medicine because they are tired of providing "hamster healthcare" and frustrated with treadmill medicine that has now become their day job.

At *Concierge Medicine Today*, we have advised and encouraged physicians, business leaders and others to remember several key points before you decide on which franchise, Concierge Medicine company or DPC consultant you select:

Do not go into debt to purchase a franchise. Downsize your lifestyle and save up and pay cash. According to one of our 2013 polls of startup concierge and DPC physicians, the majority of doctors used personal assets (savings, house, and 401K) to fund their medical venture. Financial experts encourage that, if needed, take an extra job while you are saving.

Get informed about Concierge Medicine or DPC. Talk to a number of franchisee physicians. Find out why some are struggling and others are successful. Build a relationship with your franchisor and stay in contact with them regularly. Gain as much perspective as possible before you begin. Make an educated decision.

From 2007-2012, we found the majority of private-pay practices employ less than one staff person in a Concierge Medicine clinic. These offices are often less than 2,500 square feet. Do you have leased office space that you could no longer use?

Most franchise transition companies and consultants will provide you with a Patient sales or educational support team to help you explain your new billing and services to Patients. If you have administrative or support staff that you could see coming with you, be sure they believe in where you are going and understand the new model of serving Patients. The last thing you need is your front office staff telling Patients behind your back that this is not a good deal – when in actuality, it very much is.

Many franchise, practice transition companies provide EMR, Patient/membership billing services and legal document review. Ask them what support services they provide as you plan and prepare for opening day as well as up to 9-months after your opening day.

Most importantly, look for an opportunity to evaluate the services you will enjoy providing to your Patients — not just something that offers lower risk or more money. For instance, if you are starting a Concierge Medicine or a DPC practice, ask these types of questions:

- Do I like dealing with people?
- Do I care about helping them with their healthcare needs?
- Am I more motivated by the potential money and working less hours?

Recommended Reading

Why Concierge Medicine Will Get Bigger.

Read this article at: www.ConciergeMedicineToday.com

"I finally have the time to call specialists again! I enjoy being able to interact with them more, follow up on consults, and also contact them for ongoing questions regarding Patient care. I have learned to block off about an hour per day in order to coordinate care with them. In addition, I find myself spending an hour or two on research topics during the day instead of on family time during evenings and weekends."

~Dr. Jennifer Chilek
Montgomery, TX | Stone Creek Family Medicine

"Perhaps most important from a doctors perspective," says industry consultant, Mike Permenter, whose specialty is helping doctors enter into private practice and DPC, "is that a consulting company should typically furnish all of the capital required to start or modify your medical practice and then assumes all risk for success of failure."

Companies, like MDVIP and Concierge Choice continue to capture a significant portion of the market share.

Other successful companies are operating in the marketplace: Specialdocs; Cypress Concierge Medicine; Signature MD; Latady Physician Strategies among others, continue to innovate, offering differing models, competitive transition fees and personal service to a doctors practice to help them succeed. All of these companies have an edge in that they helped build the existing industry over past years. More and more consultants and franchise-like companies like these have now come along in the past three years. They help to keep prices low and competitive, for not just their physician and clients but for satisfied Patients as well.

Specialdocs with offices in Chicago, IL and Florida states, "While we are often asked, 'what is the optimum number of Patients in a personalized care practice? The correct answer is that there is no "one size fits all" model. Each physician individually determines the appropriate number of Patients in their practice based on their ability to deliver on the promises they made to their Patients. A word of caution...even when an optimal Patient panel size is achieved, attracting new Patients will continue to be important to maintain this threshold and/or to grow the practice. Over the course of each year, all of our physician-clients experience the loss of a small number of Patients for a variety of reasons including relocation, financial setback or death. Therefore, whether you have just transitioned or have a more seasoned practice, it is important to focus on viable methods for practice growth."

Specialdocs also adds ... "Over ten years' of experience has led us to develop a "Prescription for Practice Growth." These programs include initiatives in the following areas: Interactive, Educational, Proactive Wellness and Digital Marketing. A combination of several strategies and initiatives can be used to grow a practice. Each physician needs to find his/her "marketing comfort zone" as well as what is a good fit for the community and what will provide value to their Patients."

"This new practice has been truly liberating. I am working harder than ever getting it off the ground but my time with Patients is wonderful. And I get to be creative again in how I develop the practice, something that was lost from my previous office."

-Dr. Alicia Cunningham, Vermont

"Do not start out too high." says Scott Borden of Direct Pay Consulting. "Many physicians choose Patient pricing plans that are unaffordable for most of their Patients. Remember that a higher monthly/annual membership fee will likely result in fewer Patients each with higher medical needs. Do you want to spend every day treating a few chronically ill Patients? A lower membership fee will allow healthy individuals and families that value your time to remain with your DPC practice. And you can always increase your fees next year if you completely fill your practice."

An article published by *MedScape* in July of 2013 entitled Cash-Only Practice: What You Need To Do To Succeed noted ... *because it is common for DPC practices to hemorrhage cash, at least until they attract enough Patients to pay the bills – practice managers, accountants, attorneys who actually understand healthcare law are unaffordable luxuries. As a result, and also sometimes by temperament, a lot of DPC doctors and Concierge Medicine physicians become do-it-yourselfers, often with less than optimal results.*

By now, you get the picture: the more you pay, the more brand recognition, service, technology, etc., you will get and the more operational benefits you will receive.

Mike Permenter also adds "There are a few things you should consider before joining any company. Start by asking: Is there a wide market for my concept?; What makes me different from my neighbor who is already doing this?; and Does my form of delivery [of medical care] offer a reasonable return on investment (ROI) to prospective Patients?. If the answers to questions like these is yes, then you should start the information gathering process and contact consultants and companies who can help you."

Ultimately, it all comes down to the Physician's ability to structure a program that delivers value in his/her practice. If doctors succeed in delivering value to the Patient, they are much more likely to create the win-win relationship that is the hallmark of successful business.

Medical Economics in August of 2003 wrote ... *Base your decision on your access to capital, your willingness to shoulder additional responsibilities, and you need to place your individual stamp on things.*

The Point of No Return.

You have always had something working against you when making big decisions: you. So at this point, the decision should be an easy one and you should feel comfortable with the analysis you have done and the numbers you have seen on paper. You have accounted for expenses, know what to expect and feel comfortable overcoming many of the questions and objections that people will have. It is at this time CMT/DPC Journal encourages anyone pondering a future in this marketplace to ask yourself ... 'In light of my past experiences, my current circumstances, and my future hopes and dreams [for my sanity, lifestyle, family and Patients], what is the wisest thing for me to do?'

"The conversion process is not an easy one. My staff and I are cognizant of the fact that we must consistently communicate the benefits of this choice in care, with the challenge to increase my concierge numbers and convert my non-concierge Patients," says Jeffrey S. Gorodetsky, M.D., a Concierge Doctor in Stuart, FL.

Presuming that you have found a number of loyal Patients interested in your new membership or DPC program, you will now need to explore and finalize legal issues, payor network participation, develop a service offering and work with your staff to help formulate an implementation timeline.

It is at this point doctors tell us they feel one of two emotions: fear or excitement. Where are you in this process? Are you energized about your future or scared to take the next step? If you are at a point in your evaluation process where you are still unsure, we encourage you to seek wise counsel from those smarter than you. Author and pastor, Andy Stanley says: "Wise people know when they are in no condition to decide for themselves by themselves."

This decision is emotional. But remember, emotionally charged environments are not ideal for decision-making, so it is at this point we encourage you to surround yourself with people who can see through the fog of your emotions to help you make the right decisions. Your emotions will make the obvious less obvious. This is why you are probably better at managing someone else's health rather than your own. It is why you know exactly what your Patient needs to do about their health, but lack insight that you need to improve your own. When it comes to making this decision, remember that it is next to impossible to hear the voice of wisdom when emotions are raging. You should consider inviting someone or multiple someone's into your area of weakness and listen to them. Let them see what you cannot see.

Franchising can be a tremendously advantageous — and fast — way of expanding your medical practice into the area of Concierge Medicine or DPC. This is particularly true for the doctor who lacks the time, manpower and the finances to open a practice alone. It is a strategy that works even during times of economic uncertainty.

"Becoming a concierge physician is an opportunity to give my patients the special personal touch that they like, need, and desire! The concierge practice will afford me the opportunity to engage my patients about all aspects of their healthcare: preventative, social, family, fitness & wellness, as well as nutrition, and all the while spending a good deal of quality time with them.
For physicians, concierge practice is our chance to practice medicine the way it was before insurance companies started dictating healthcare.
I am very excited about the opportunity for my patients as well as myself."
-Dr. Eddie Richardson, Eatonton, GA

D.I.Y.

Consultants, Franchise Opportunities & Team Approach: Pros, Cons and Costs.

"You really have to plan that it is truly going to take you several months to a year to get up and running," says Catherine Jordan, MSA, RN, LNCC, a legal nurse consultant who advises at VantagePoint.

Hiring the expertise you need can be costly. Many consultants advise physicians to have significant cash reserves available to operate the practice before a Concierge Medicine or DPC practice conversion is ever considered. A practice manager who not only knows their stuff but whom Patients like is a must, as is a good accountant and trusted attorney who understands local healthcare laws for your state. Tax lawyers are typically not recommended.

Currently, there is a phenomenal opportunity for doctors to innovate and move into the Concierge Medicine or DPC space.

When you purchase a franchised business, you are paying for two things. First, you are paying for a proven system. You are stepping into a business plan and a company that likely has been around awhile and has a proven track-record of financial success. The second thing a franchise offers is a national or recognizable brand. For example, MDVIP is instantly recognizable in the Concierge Medicine and private-pay medical marketplace as one of those national brands.

Franchises are a very popular method of entering the Concierge Medicine or DPC marketplace for some doctors. It allows physicians to change, start and even grow a unique medical practice while at the same time learning from the experts in place with a proven track record to help you. One of the biggest advantages of joining a franchise Concierge Medicine or DPC medical care group is that you have access to an established company's brand name; meaning later on, you do not have to spend additional resources to get your name and services out to Patients.

Generally speaking, franchising means opening additional outlets through the sale of franchise rights to independent physicians who will use the Company's name and system of operations. A franchisee pays a franchisor an initial franchise fee in return for the rights to operate a practice under the franchise trademark and name and for training in how to operate the business.

Levels of operational and marketing support vary between franchising organizations. Be sure to find out exactly what is offered and included before signing on the dotted line. For many doctors, franchising can be the ideal form of business expansion. Some preliminary questions may include: One of the most common questions physicians ask when exploring this private-pay medical marketplace for the first-time is 'how much does it cost to transition my insurance-based medical practice to this new DPC or retainer-based business model?'

- Who owns the Patient Contracts?
- Do prospective Patients call you or my office directly?
- How much support is offered during the transition process?
- Do you place staff in my office? If so, permanently or just during the transition process?
- What type of technology (if any) will you bring to my office?
- What about my staff?
- Can I speak to the last 5 doctors who joined the franchise? Preferably within the past 6 to 12 months?
- What marketing support is provided during the conversion process?
- After conversion what type of marketing support will you provide?
- What training do you provide?
- How are your fees structured? Multi-year residuals?
- Is corporate restructuring needed?
- What type of support (if any) is provided should the number of Patients converted not meet our target?
- How are referrals handled?
- Do you have discounted relationships with imaging centers, labs, etc.?
- What legal support is provided?
- Can I speak to a doctor who has been with you 3-5 years in a similar market?
- What are my options at the end of our contract term?
- What are the early opt-out provisions?
- What if I sell my practice? Retire?

These are just a few of the questions you want to ask in the very early stages of investigating joining a franchise. Add to them the unique questions posed by your current practice. Talk to at least 2-3 consultants and/or franchisors prior to making your decisions. Be sure to check references!

Franchise and consulting fees can move from five-figures and easily into six figures. *Concierge Medicine Today* found the average cost is between $150,000 – $250,000 over a period of two to five years and, in some rare cases, even longer. Some consultants have quoted figures less than $60,000. Depending on your practice, demographics, your bedside manner, Patient surveys (very important), complexity of internal operations in a practice, a financial feasibility analysis, and a number of other variables, that will determine whether a Concierge Medicine or DPC practice is the right option for you.

As with most of the companies operating in the concierge medical marketplace, a doctor (i.e. franchisee) will pay an ongoing periodic royalty fee. We found this to be as low as 15% of each Patient's individual membership fee. However in most cases, it is between 29% to 33% for a period of approximately 3 to 5 years. In some rare cases, up to 25% of your per Patient fee for eight years has been reported by doctors considering a career in Concierge Medicine or DPC. These fees usually include continued support and training in advertising: marketing; sales; operational guidance; technology; legal; regulatory; financial and human resources consulting; and other services.

Important Next Steps.

In this book we have listed a detailed description of the Pros and Cons of the various business models and payment structures. Now it is time to start preparing internally for some big changes, some tough questions and a great deal of curiosity about your new practice approach from Patients, family members, friends, colleagues and the media.

Before you begin, remember, there is no wrong choice. It is about what business model and decision works best for you, your Patients, your lifestyle and quality of life, your family, your local demographic and Patient population. Now that you have the facts, you are probably leaning toward one model for your practice versus another. So decide now which model is your best choice.

Once you have chosen a business model, it is time to assemble a team, find a consultant or maybe meet with your staff and discuss some of the changes ahead. Here are some additional items to start thinking about as you move forward.

Develop a Timeline

Moving your practice from a traditional, managed care, insurance reliant practice to a Concierge Medicine practice is a labor intensive process. It will take time and a lot of planning. A timeline, complete with goals and objectives will help keep you focused and moving forward if designed thoroughly and early in the planning phase. Follow it, and your road to success will be easier and much more likely.

Address Legal Issues In Your State, Talk To A Trusted Healthcare Attorney.

We have already discussed some of the obvious legal challenges to starting a Concierge Medicine practice. It is the advice of countless physicians that you find a trusted attorney who understands your states: healthcare laws, new practice structure; service offering(s); Medicare participation; insurer contracts; the Affordable Care Act (ACA), etc. If you are unable to locate of find a Concierge Medicine or DPC attorney, www.ConciergeMedicineToday.com has a list of resources that you can use to help get you started.

Explain The Practice To Insurers

Generally, insurance companies and local health plans will not prohibit physicians from opening Concierge Medicine, retainer-based or DPC practices. Susan Pisano, a spokesperson for the American Association of Health Plans told Medical Economics in an interview that insurers will still cover contractually obligated practice and hospital-based services and procedures. The fee a Concierge Medicine doctor charges should be for "extras" like monitoring specialist care, enhanced access, etc., if a Patient ends up in a hospital. At the same time, it is important to be very cautious in your communication and conversations with health insurers in your state. "Many want to look at marketing materials to confirm that what plan members are paying are for extra time and attention, not covered medical services," said Allison McCarthy, consultant at Corporate Health Group in a story to Medical Economics. She tells the writer to be ready to share whatever materials you have and make any reasonable changes that are called for.

Additional considerations which we will address in more detail later in the book also include:

- Addressing FAQs and Educating Your Staff
- Use of Your Current EMR/EHR capabilities in Your New Business Model Design
- Billing Procedures To Patients (i.e. quarterly; monthly; annually, etc.)

Crafting Your Message. Should I Hire Someone Or Pay A Company To Do My Marketing?

Create Marketing Materials:

Education and messaging when venturing into the marketplace and communications to Patients are critical. When you reach out to your Patients, regardless of age, experts say the key is to promote a new corporate image. An image that is consistent with the enhanced level of services you are going to offer. That may mean a new lead-generating web site, logo, business cards, letterhead, email address and possibly even a new corporate name.

Just so there is no confusion, marketing and crafting your message is a big part of your next step forward. You need to take the time to carefully craft and perfect the message(s) you are going to be sending to Patients.

There is help out there and you should know how to use it. What doctors tell us is that they wish they would have hired a smart public relations and Patient advocate with a strong marketing background to help them write and communicate clear messages to their Patients. What doctors know now that they did not know when they started is that there is a big difference between the services provided by a 'marketing consultant' versus an 'advertising firm.'

"Really competent advertisers have a better handle on the pulse of the culture than anybody else." notes Rush Limbaugh in a recent discussion about advertising during a recent radio program. "It is their job. They have one job: Separate people from their money, willingly. Their job is to convince John Q. Public to give up his money for whatever they convince John Q. Public he wants."

Limbaugh continues, "I have always believed that if a company hires an agency to sell its product -- to market and sell its product -- that agency has to know the culture. That agency has to know what is cool, it has to know what is hip, and it has to be able to predict it [behavior], and it has to be able to personify it [the brand]. It also has to be able to hire people who can write and produce it [ads]. There are all kinds of different advertising. There is cost per thousand, there is results oriented, and there is impressions, any number of ways of going about it. Television advertising in the Super Bowl is a combination of cost per thousand reaching eyeballs, but also results oriented and branding. For example, prime time [television], you watch any show that is targeting the 25-54 demographic, and you will learn what those people think is cool, hip, and where our culture is. If you watch the Super Bowl and really take time to watch the commercials and study them rather than be entertained by them, you will find out you will have a pretty good bead on where the country is culturally."

"The 55-plus hasn't been abandoned," adds Limbaugh. "But the advertising aimed at them is simply aimed at maintaining brand loyalty and establishing that the products they love are still good and still work and maybe are being improved. But you will not see advertising aimed at those people that is designed to get them to switch brands. The advertising aimed at 25-54 is all about that. And, by the way, not every advertising agency knows what it is doing. That is why some are better than others. It is like any other business, some Super Bowl commercials, you say, "What the bleep was that?" Utter failure, if that is your reaction."

As you move forward with the announcement of your Concierge Medicine, DPC or membership program in your practice, you need to know which one is right for you. Marketing Consultants will generally advise you and help to develop your strategy and plan whereas advertising agencies will execute the agreed upon plan for you. If you do not have the staff resources to effectively execute the strategy you may want to consider using an ad agency or ca consultant who advises **and** executes your plan.

Remember, these are two very different types of consultants that can and should be helping you building your Concierge Medicine or DPC communication plan. A Marketing Consultant should have marketplace expertise or have access to resources to both write and design materials and effective, lead-generating communications for your practice. Some medical practices hire marketing representatives and bring them on board as employees to represent the practice.

Marketing or ad agencies typically offer both offline and online advertising strategies to grow your Patient-base and be able to outline a plan that works with your budget. They are typically paid by the project or will quote you prices for the services that you wish for them to perform.

Which one is better? Physicians and healthcare practices tell us that budgeting money and giving it to a marketing agency or ad firm is the most effective strategy of growing a medical practice. More often than not, an internal marketing person or employee you have hired will naturally take on daily tasks and duties put onto them by the doctor or staff that is not part of their job description. Over time, staff find that a marketing person or "employee" of a medical practice is not as effective as they had hoped because they are paying a salary to this person who is now not fully dedicated to the marketing of the practice, plus, the marketing and promotional task expenses.

Pricing Your Service Competitively

We have talked to, surveyed and collected data from over 1,000 confirmed, currently operating concierge practices in the U.S. in 2012 and 2013. Through this process, we have determined the national average annual fee for concierge medical services is between $1,400-$2,000 per Patient, per year. Large networks of Concierge Doctors have claimed a significant portion of the Concierge Doctor market share and thus help to keep prices from inflating too high in major metropolitan markets.

In addition, we found that some independent Concierge Doctors who are not part of a large group charge higher rates ($2,500 and up).

Interviews with various industry sources indicate that the average Patient or consumer of concierge medical services market can withstand a small annual premium increase of about $25 to $160 per year. The problem with raising prices for concierge Patients, especially in private, DPC medicine and concierge medical clinics is that it causes Patients to reassess how much value this care brings to their life, including their financial commitment, their current quality of life, past experiences with the doctors' staff, traffic and travel interruptions and how often they actually utilize services on an annual basis.

We receives inquiries every day from Patients looking to join a Concierge Medicine or DPC practice. We routinely receive inquiries from doctors who are looking at how much they are charging for services. They are attempting to determine how they can balance those fees and still charge what their Patients will pay without appearing to price-gouge their Patients.

"*If you possess excellent communication skills, around the clock dedication and the desire to promote optimal health in pursuit of excellent medicine, then Concierge Medicine is for you. It is the best career choice I have ever made.*"

-Brian Thornburg, MSM, DO, PA, FAAP
Innovative Pediatrics, Florida

Instill Passion In Your Staff For Your "Concierge" Practice Model

"I promised my staff that they would have better lives, better working conditions, they would all get raises, and none of them would be let go, ..." ~Dr. Thomas LaGrelius, Torrance, CA

We have spoken to numerous Concierge Medicine and DPC doctors from different parts of the country that tell the same story ... *'I had an employee who didn't believe in my medical practice model and they were telling Patients to go somewhere else. I should have done something but They have been with me for years.'*

One of the main reasons why Patients leave their concierge physician is often due to the fact that they do not like your staff. That's right. Passionate employees produce better results – but keeping someone who has been loyal to you for years but you know deep down is not good for business can cause more harm than good to your bottom line. The best way to spark passion in your front office employees, nurses and other staff is to demonstrate your own passion — but do not be a cheerleader at staff meetings. Here are some simple ways to authentically show your enthusiasm and inspire others:

Have everyone share a success story once a month at your staff meeting.

This will help build camaraderie among your staff as well as lasting memories that help foster the kind of stories that you and your staff want to achieve from month-to-month.

Focus on the positive.

Author and business consultant Marcus Buckingham wrote a book about this. He writes ... *Unfortunately, most of us have little sense of our talents and strengths, much less the ability to build our lives around them. Instead, guided by our parents, by our teachers, by our managers, and by psychology's fascination with pathology, we become experts in our weaknesses and spend our lives trying to repair these flaws, while our strengths lie dormant and neglected.* Too often we focus on the bad thing(s) that went wrong. While this is necessary to discuss at times in your business, we need to learn as managers of businesses to encourage and help employees grow and use their strengths at work. Employees know when a doctor truly cares about his or her practice. Passionate Concierge Medicine doctors cannot help but talk about what is working well and try to find ways to fix what is not. So, help your employees nurture their strengths month-to-month — you will be glad you did!

Set goals and expectations. One of the reasons that mega-churches are growing so fast across the U.S. is that they have set expectations with their audience week in and week out. It is no different in a doctor's office. You should know exactly what to expect when you walk in. You should know whether you are going to be greeted with a smile, an ill-tempered staff member that needs to find another job or you will be given a bill. Which scenario sounds best to you?

This does not mean unattainable workloads. Passionate concierge physician entrepreneurs should inspire and challenge their employees to do their best, without overloading them. A great tip is to break your goals and expectations into little tiny goals creating easy wins for your team. This constant state of winning will be a guaranteed formula for success. Everyone wants to be with the winning team. Success breeds success and it is infectious.

Encourage everyone on your staff to be part of the relational, healthy lifestyle process.

I believe that in order for sustained, healthy lifestyle change to occur, we have to grow together with those whom we have surrounded ourselves. This happens best inside a doctor's office when together, Patients, employees and the doctor(s) are prioritizing intentional relationships and all are seeking the same goal. Walked out, this means that if a Patient is struggling with a weight problem, broken their arm or coping with a more serious chronic condition, they want to know that it is not just the doctor who cares — but the receptionist on my way out who asks me if I am okay too.

Hiring Concierge/DPC Medical Staff Using Job Descriptions With Performance Standards For Key Measurement

Whether we like it or not, Concierge Medicine offices and DPC clinics are held to a higher standard of service and performance, not just by our colleagues who are either pessimistic or optimistic and curious, but by Patients who are now expecting something different from you, your facility and of course, your entire staff. Performance standards for your employees inside your Concierge Medicine offices or DPC should form the heart of their job description. Make sure their job description describes the what is, how-to's, and how-wells of a job for employees in this new service business.

Each of your performance standards should state three things about the employee's job:

- What the employee is to do;
- When they are to do it;
- How it is to be done; and
- To what extent it is to be done (how much, how well, how soon).

A business owner can use a good job description not only as a valuable aid in the recruiting and hiring process, but also as a list of the duties and responsibilities for what the employee is to do for Patients and in your practice each day while on the job. A job description using performance standards is <u>much</u> more useful than a simple explanation of duties or qualifications.

'I'd actually be happy to pay an extra $199 or even more for a real improvement. And if my current doctor switched to a concierge practice model I'd go with her and pay more. But the concierge model as a whole has a lot to prove before it really catches on.'

-MedCity News, January 2014

Anatomy of a Concierge Medical Staff Performance Standard

- **Job classification:** Front Office Manager
- **Type of work:** Scheduling, records updates, phone calls, and public relations with Patients
- **Performance Standard:** The Front Office Manager will cheerfully help Patients when they arrive and answer questions with 100% accuracy using our internal standard of business procedures.
- **How this looks on a day-to-day basis:** The Front Office Manager may encounter the following and will ...

Mary Massad, Director of HR Product Development for Insperity (previously known as Administaff, Inc.) says "When it comes to job descriptions, flexibility is the key. It may be wise to create more generic job descriptions that emphasize expectations and accountabilities, rather than specific tasks, thereby encouraging employees to focus on results rather than job duties."

Better work means better productivity, better customer service, more sales, higher profits and happy Patients. Once workers know what to do and how to do it, they can concentrate on improving their skills. Improved skills and knowledge, coupled with goals to be met, encourage people to work more independently.

Morale in your practice is important. A performance standard system can reduce conflict and misunderstanding in your practice as well. Everybody knows who is responsible for what. They know what parts of the job are most important. They know the level of performance you expect in each job.

Consistent use of a performance standard system can not only reduce or eliminate low productivity, it can reduce high turnover. When your employees are told clearly what to do and you have set expectations early, they are shown what to do on the job, in writing. They now know what is expected and have a way to determine how well they are doing on a daily, monthly or quarterly basis because there is a standard of measurement which you can use to monitor their effectiveness in that position. As a physician, you can also help and support them with additional continuing development education and programs including conferences, seminars, training or service coaching. This can be particularly helpful when the standards are not being met as you'd like in the practice. The investment in your employees can and generally will pay off over time through increased knowledge, skills and attitude. All this makes for much better relationships between you and your employees.

"Direction, not intention determines your destination."

— Andy Stanley, Author/Pastor

Chapter 5 –
Public Introduction, Part 1.
Learn, Listen & Discover.

Dramatic Decision-Making.

The riskiest 10 to 18 weeks for any business especially those in the Concierge Medicine and private medical marketplace is when it first opens. In the first two years, three of every ten startups go out of business according to the US Small Business Administration (SBA). We have surveyed doctors over the past several years and have found that 10% of doctors starting a concierge or retainer-based practice go out of business in the first two years also. While the US SBA also claims that by five years, half of those startups are history, the Concierge Medicine and direct care industry is still so new, we cannot confirm with certainty that this statistic applies.

Getting Your Concierge Medicine or DPC Practice Past Year One (1).

The Tactical Approach. 19 Steps To Ensure A Smooth Road Ahead.

So how can you improve the odds that your practice startup will survive that tough first year? We have sifted through countless interview notes and sought out expertise from industry consultants, physicians and their staff to help you succeed. Here are a few important steps to take:

1. **Do You Need Additional Help With Your Transition Or Can You Resource In-House?**

   Most medical offices are simply too busy to handle the complexities of the transition themselves. According to *Concierge Medicine Today* over half of physicians across the U.S. state that they used a consultant of some sort to aid in their transition process. Albeit, a local practice management consultant in the area they knew or a more formal, experienced company operating in the Concierge Medicine marketplace, the majority of doctors recognized they needed help. Further, they are glad they did.

2. **Technology, EMR and Billing.**

   Industry consultants recommend that doctors not implement a new EMR or electronic health record (EHR) system of any kind during the 3 month to 6-month transition period.

Adding the advanced learning curve of technology to staff responsibilities, and your own, is simply an unwise idea. Should you need to re-tool or update some of your office systems, experts say, you need a system that will enable you to track the status of your former Patients (I.e. those who chose not to participate in your new practice or program and who may have switched to another doctor due to your recent practice changes. The system should also monitor which Patients are current Patients and manage the appointments and communicate often and regularly with your new ones. A number of programs are coming out to assist doctors with their technology needs
Review them carefully to choose the best one for your practice.

3. **When Will Patients Pay You? Will You Accept Credit Cards From Your Patients?**

A few years back we conducted a survey to find out the percentage of Concierge Medicine doctors who did or did not accept credit card payments from their Patients. At the time, we found that approximately 51% of Concierge Medical doctors gave their Patients this option or were looking into adding it. This percentage is obviously on the increase. We will update the percentage of credit card participation as it becomes available.

In this section, we felt it was important to find out how often Concierge Medicine Patients pay their doctor the annual fee. With the advent of simple and low cost options for doctors and clinic owners to allow their Patients to swipe their cards to pay their checks – we wanted to know if Patients were paying their Concierge Doctor monthly, quarterly or annually.

The data *Concierge Medicine Today* learned was:

- 42% of Patients Pay Monthly.
- 21% of Patients Pay Quarterly.
- 36% of Patients Pay Annual/One-Time.

In December 2013, we reported that January 2014 would kick-off the most significant month in the industry's growth, a Tipping Point. Most people sign up in January through March of each year. September is also a popular month each year for Concierge Medicine membership program enrollment.

4. **Decide What You Can Afford.**

Most Concierge Medicine practices report that they are able to reduce overhead and operational expenses dramatically in the first six to eighteen months, according to interviews by *Concierge Medicine Today*. Look for every possible way to save. This will allow you to keep going longer, hopefully until revenue starts to cover your practice expenses.

We routinely tell doctors that once you are up and running, the ideal overhead of a lean office is approximately 30% of your gross revenue. The breakdown of overhead should be

50% for staff and consultants 25%-30% for recent and utilities and the remaining 25% for miscellaneous expenses (office supplies, insurance, prescription cost, machine maintenance, and advertising).

Although concierge medical clinics and DPC doctors' offices are popping up across the country, some hopeful owners are still struggling to get financing. This has many "docpreneurs" wondering how to go about getting the cash they need to either start or maintain their medical business. Postpone unnecessary purchases, or pick up a broom and clean the office yourself. Surveys from physicians and their staff tell us that the majority of Concierge Medicine and DPC practices employ less than 2 employees.

5. **Plan for Problems.**

The only thing as sure as death and taxes is that unexpected issues will crop up with your newly born private-pay, concierge medical business. Sit down and think about everything that could go wrong – then, make a plan for how you will survive each possible scenario. Talking with an attorney prior to having someone take legal action is and could be a very important step for your practice to survive in the years ahead.

6. **Draft a Continuity of Care Letter With A Trusted Attorney.**

Continuity of care is an important part of Patient relations, particularly as it relates to communicating with insured Patients who no longer wish to visit or participate in your practice. Some insurance plans will take immediate action to protect the care of their members, so be sure you work with an attorney to help draft this document to ensure compliance with State laws, Medicare, etc.

Most, if not all, Concierge Medicine and DPC physician offices help coordinate all continuation of care for their Patients who choose to no longer participate or visit the practice. Some doctors provide a list of doctors in the area accepting new Patients, their contact number, specialist referrals, etc. To avoid frustration among your colleagues, it is advised by industry consultants that your practice contact these offices prior to referring a large number of Patients to them within a small period of time. Communication between primary care physicians and specialists is crucial to your Patients and of the utmost importance to health plans. Make sure you do this step correctly and seek the counsel of a good attorney.

7. **Should I Send A Letter To My Colleagues?**
   If So, About What And Why?

Q: A physician asked us, "Would sending a letter to some of my colleagues, maybe outside my specialty, which is located in my area, help me acquire new Patients?"

Answer: Yes! Physicians at a recent conference focused on this topic a lot. It does work. The first thing you want to do is collect a list of the practitioner's names and addresses in your area. Address the letter to them personally (i.e. the doctor), thank them for reading your letter (this might sound weird ... but it works, so be sure to include it). Try to solve their problems. What value and services would their Patients have by coming to see you?

Last, state near the end of the letter that 'you eagerly anticipate collaborating with them in the very near future. You might even want to ask them questions also. For example, what type of Patients do you treat or would like for your practice to refer to them? Are they comfortable handling Medicare Patients? etc.

8. **Choose your location carefully.**

    Whether you are in a town where Patients can see your practice on public streets or one where you will be located in a suite of offices, make sure your practice is conveniently located and accessible to maximize "new" prospective Patient interest.

9. **Analyze your numbers.**

    Even though it is hard to find time in those crazy days after you first start signing up Patients, it is important to stop and look at your numbers to see where your practice is headed. With 10% of concierge and private-pay medical practices folding in the first two years, it is vital to understand and forecast where your greatest potential is to grow your practice. If your practice is not going where you would like it to, change course and surround yourself with good advisers, even other physicians in similar situations and medical practices can help. Most successful concierge medical practices go through multiple internal process changes before they find what works for their practice.

10. **Sending A Notification Letter To Patients.**

Your Patients already know, like and trust you. This is key to your success. It is, by and large, why this endeavor will work. It is critical that your message is one of caring when you formulate your letter to announce to Patients that you are moving into Concierge Medicine, a DPC or a membership medicine style practice model. You will want to be sure to explain to Patients in one page or less, that this change will benefit their health and their ease of access when seeking medical care at your practice. Be sure to include a firm date for response and your practice transition. Just about every physician who has crafted this letter to send to their Patients advises others to keep it brief and highlight the features and benefits of the practice – not a diatribe from the doctor about insurance carrier reimbursements or ethical issues he/she has with the Affordable Care Act. This is not the place to vent your personal opinion(s). That is what blogs are for.

Keep the letter brief and to the point, invite Patients to call for more information and keep the communication positive. There is no one magical template here that will recruit every Patient. This is designed to educate your Patients and compel a response, positive or negative. Even the most well-crafted writers and most talented doctors and marketing staff will not be able to win over everyone. Your goal with this communication is to provide them with answers to their questions in the most friendly, accommodating and educational way possible.

11. **Talk to Your Patients, Early and Often.**

Your patients will have questions, particularly the ones that really want to join. They are going to ask, "How does this work with my current insurance?" The doctor, staff and nurses employed at your practice are going to need to have an answer for this as well as other difficult questions. Included in this Guidebook is a list of FAQs and the answers to help you. This is found on page 133.

12. **Plan, Both Formal and Informal, Educational Sign-Up Meetings.**

An activity that is most often overlooked is the use of informational meetings inside your practice with a small group of Patients. These would be in addition to more formal and larger, planned events designed to educate the uninformed Patient base about upcoming changes. Each of these types of meetings should involve the doctor answering some of the most FAQs your Patients may have about the letter or invitation they received. These events should put you, the physician, up close and personal with prospective enrollees and Patients. Agendas should be planned ahead of time by you and your staff (or consultant) and should educate and enhance the image of your new program or practice. These events should also be designed to create top of mind awareness (TOMA) with prospective Patients.

One of the main reasons that these events are overlooked is because doctors do not know how or where to begin. The second is, it takes time. Usually someone in the practice, often the Office Manager, must spend a few hours each month on the phone making connections and inviting current and former Patients to these meetings.

Industry consultants explain that if the Physician is upfront and personal with the invited Patients, they can enroll as many as twenty (20%) percent of attendees into the new practice or membership medicine program. The investment you will make in these formal and informal educational events is not always monetary. It simply costs the Physician's time and the time of someone employed by the practice. The doctor should be heavily involved in the presentation and planning of the meetings. Having the Physician take the lead role in the presentation to Patients will make the return on investment (ROI) even greater. The Physician should attend all of these meetings to create a face to go with the name and brand of the practice or new program. After all, Concierge Medicine's mission is about access to the Doctor. How would it look it they are not there or choose not to participate in the presentation and explanation of benefits to their Patients and prospective enrollees?

13. **Create Your Own Community Events.**

Your local community is your livelihood. Inviting local churches, local businesses, Rotary

Members, Optimist Club and other such business networking clubs in the area in which you participate is an excellent way to attract new Patients into your practice.

Another way community events are facilitated to become a real, operating marketing activity in your practice is to create your own event(s) each quarter. This might involve a partnership with a charity during the holidays or declare a month "Fiber In Your Diet Awareness Month," "Nutrition Check-Up Month," etc. This is where you can be creative and encourage your staff to participate. These events can drive former and current Patients to join your practice and create positive word of mouth advertising.

14.   **Use Routine Follow-Up Appointments To Your Advantage.**

As previously indicated, the Doctor is truly the best person to answer the Patient's questions. After all, isn't that why you are moving into this space? Do not avoid the questions your Patients ask by relying on your staff to answer those questions. That is one of the worst reactions Doctors can have, advise currently practicing concierge and DPC doctors. If you rely on your staff to address the difficult questions about your new program before or after their exam room visit with you, you have missed the opportunity to recruit that Patient face-to-face. The Patient will be reluctant and skeptical and probably not sign up for what you are selling and promoting.

15.   **Media Training, The Press and Sending Press Releases.**

In the book, *The Marketing MD* by Michael Tetreault, sending out press releases is a great way to get picked up by local news sites and blogs that people actually read. These allow you to position yourself as a dependable resource and medical professional with your local media. You might not believe you have anything newsworthy to contribute, but you would be surprised just how much your opinion is needed in the media today.

The Marketing MD book recommends you market yourself as a resource on specific topics, such as: nutrition; diabetes; general pediatric; or internal medicine topics; or on specific issues about which you have unique expertise. Both local broadcasting stations and the print media are excellent forums for you to use in getting your name known in the community as an expert physician.

If you choose to take your press release and thought online, The Marketing MD book recommends that you use web sites that will link back to your web site. By doing this, the book states, you can increase your ranking on Google. The book also provides a long list of recommended press release sites you can use. *The Marketing MD* book is available at www.ConciergeMedicineToday.com.

16. **Dealing With Unhappy Concierge Medicine Patients and Using Comment Cards.**

Patients do not speak with their mouths, they speak with their feet as well as quietly on the

Internet, sometimes known as 'the coward's canvas.' Typically, when your Patients are unhappy, they simply do not come back. Why? It could be a bad attitude, unprofessional service, a price increase or a change in the physical location of your practice. Most Concierge Medicine Doctors may never know. But one thing is for certain, allowing your Patients an avenue to express their concerns indirectly through the use of comment or suggestion cards can help you keep your Patients year after year. With the national Concierge Medicine Patient retention rate slipping from 94 percent in 2010, 92 percent in 2012 and now 91% in 2014, it is more important than ever to maintain your current Patient base.

According to one recent national poll of currently practicing Concierge Medicine and DPC doctors, we found that it takes on average between three to four months to acquire one new Patient to a Concierge Medicine practice. Additional digging by the same source also revealed that it can cost three times more to acquire a new Patient than to keep an existing Patient happy. Therefore, a well-executed Patient Comment Card system and drop box by your door, in your lobby or in any place where a Patient has to wait for you — gives you the vital information you need at the end of the day and shows that you respect the time, opinion and comments of your current Patients. Not to mention, it also offers a simple, hassle-free way to give feedback to your staff — good and bad.

Encourage your Patients to fill-in the card completely by giving incentives such as a complimentary $5 gift card on their next visit. Birthday and anniversary ideas are also great incentives too. "One of the best Patient incentives I received was a hand-written congratulations card from my doctor when I graduated from business school with my MBA," said one University of Georgia graduate school and Patient of a Concierge Doctor. "I may have mentioned it in passing but I never in a million years thought my doctor cared."

You do not need to spend big bucks on mass mailer or a local newspaper ad to attract new Patients. While those items should be part of your marketing plan, comment cards focus on keeping the Patients who already know, like and trust you and hopefully, value the services you provide to them.

You will increase frequency of existing Patients simply by asking these questions and offering a "thank-you" gift to be redeemed at a future date. Work with your marketing team and staff to create fun redemptions. If you think you need legal advice, run the incentive or gift past your attorney for about 5 minutes.

Be creative. Design a comment card (with a drop box too – do not rely on people to hand it to your staff) that people will want to complete. Include a section for rating the doctor on today's visit, staff service, wait time, if any, office setting, and additional comments.

The last section should ask for more basic information. Here's where you can start building a valuable database, e.g. birthdays, anniversary, children's birthdays, etc.

Last and equally as important. If something goes wrong in your Concierge Medicine or DPC practice, you want to have the chance to make it right—right away. Do not let that Patient walk away from your practice for good.

Email us at editor@conciergemedicinetoday.com and we'll send you the PDF Patient Comment Card template for FREE for adaption into your practice.

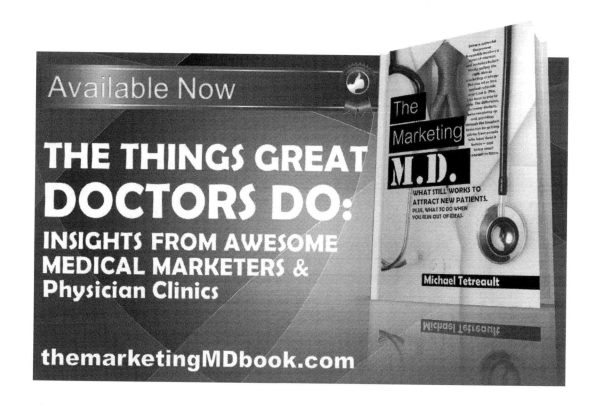

17. **Ask The Patient For Their Advice.** This is a simple action that can really make you and your employees look like you care about the service you provide ... and you do, right? The Patient has an opinion if you will simply ask them ... 'did we take care of all your needs today?' Asking your Patients for their opinion and they will share it with you. It could be the best question you ever asked and result in a Patient referral or another year or month of membership from someone who was thinking about cancelling their membership with your medical practice until you simply listened to them that day.

The most important thing for a Concierge Medicine or DPC practice to remember is to always be friendly, courteous, helpful, and professional. By keeping these tips in mind, you and your staff can avoid big blunders and keep you from losing Patients.

18. **Get "Social." Use Your Staff To Help.**

As many businesses and private medical doctors' fight for the attention of customers and Patients in order to get a positive revenue stream in place over the next 12 months, there are a number of ways to go about securing your place in the hearts and minds of local Patients.

Whether you have chosen to promote your concierge or DPC medical practice through traditional "offline" advertising methods such as printed materials in the form of postcards, Patient referral and appointment cards, brochures, etc., keep some of these "online" ideas in mind in 2015:

> **Promote through your employees.** Even though your workers have enough to do on a daily basis, they are on the front line in your practice and probably interact with them quite often. Therefore, it only makes sense to have them promote your medical practice through pictures, spoken word or testimonial. Your employees can do such things as spread the word to their family and friends through Facebook, Pinterest, Instagram or Twitter; along with assisting you in your social media promotions agenda. If you choose this route, make sure your staff knows your policy toward social media. No HIPPA violations or pictures of Patients or private documents – among other privacy concerns. When trying to save money on your advertising/marketing/promotional budgets each year, turn to your workers to help spread the word.

> **Place A Strong Emphasis On Social Media And Email.** If 2014 or the past year saw you giving minimal or no effort towards social media, by all means change that over the next 12 months. While some doctors still do not see the value in social media and they feel they cannot see a clear return on investment (ROI), most of your Patients (and employees) actively still engage in it every day. So, if you have had little interaction with your medical practice's Facebook, Twitter, Google+, Pinterest and other social media pages, make a change quickly and start informing your Patients of local news, healthier recipes you have tried, photos and more about your practice. Jump on your social media pages about 20-minutes a day (according to the book *Facebook Marketing For Doctors: 20-Minutes A Day*) and provide your audience relevant information that will

answer questions your current Patients and prospective Patients may have and help them with issues to which you have the answers.

19. The Glass Window Effect.

It is often been examined and criticized that having two entrances for your Patients if you are a Concierge Doctor is elitist and rude. While this opinion may have some fans, from a customer service and Patient relations perspective, it is sometimes necessary to have two entrances that have two lobby/check-in desks but it is never acceptable, from a Patient service point-of-view, to have a glass window [i.e. barrier] between you and a Concierge Medicine Patient.

If you participate in a Concierge Medicine practice that accepts insurance and has a concierge program, here's the problem with one entrance in some concierge medical clinics – you still have one entrance for all your Patients.

Let me explain. When you have one entrance and lobby for all of your Patients, there is usually a check-in desk or glass window. Logistically and for HIPAA reasons this is understandable, and when these Patients arrive you'd like to know whether or not they are an insured Patient or on the concierge program, right? Well, this might sound fine from an operational standpoint, but put yourself in the position of the concierge Patient.

If I'm paying a premium to see my doctor, you better know my name when I arrive and I sure shouldn't have to tap on the glass when I walk-in. This sends the wrong message to Patients about your customer service. You will see it reflected in your Patient retention when it comes time for those Concierge Medicine program Patients to renew their membership or subscription with your practice.

Making The Case for Concierge Care and Your New Practice Model.

Until recently, primary care and most health care practices were one of the only businesses in America that rarely listed how much they charged for services and products. The eventual evolution of concierge healthcare business models changed all of that.

Concierge Medicine's Best Kept Secret, the Price.

Concierge Medicine makes up a small but growing percentage of medical practices. However, if there is one thing learned in the past several years about Concierge Medicine, it is that people really do not understand how many Doctors there are and that it is not healthcare for the rich. We should think of these pioneering doctors who carry around a medical bag with a stethoscope inside who come to the aid of our family and our bedside as visionary physicians who want to normalize their practices, getting back to practicing medicine as it was before 1960.

DPC Clinics Take Cue From Retail With Greater Customer Focus.

As the healthcare system prepares to cope with an influx of the estimated 30 million Americans who will ultimately have health coverage as a result of the Affordable Care Act, a surging market of DPC (DPC) and retail clinics are poised to take on a wider role to relieve the bottleneck.

"Instead of viewing the status quo PCP model as the center of the universe," says Dr. Robert Nelson, a DPC physician based in Georgia. "Maybe we should take some plays from the Retail Clinic playbook before we become obsolete."

The Cost of Concierge Medicine In America.

We believe if more people are exposed to the cost value of Concierge and DPC medical care, it will make a big difference on what they spend. A recent story in *The New York Times* supports this belief. The paper reports that the State of Indiana offers a high-deductible plan and another that is a traditional HMO. People in the high-deductible plan spend thousands less than those in the HMO.

"The average expense in 2009 for Patients on one of these [high-deductible] plans was $6,393," the paper writes, "compared with $8,570 for Patients enrolled in a more traditional health maintenance organization plan."

Furthermore, many Concierge Physicians offer access to wholesale pricing through negotiated discounts on prescriptions, lab tests, imaging services and medical supplies for pennies on the dollar, like Dr. Chris Ewin of 121MD in Fort Worth, TX.

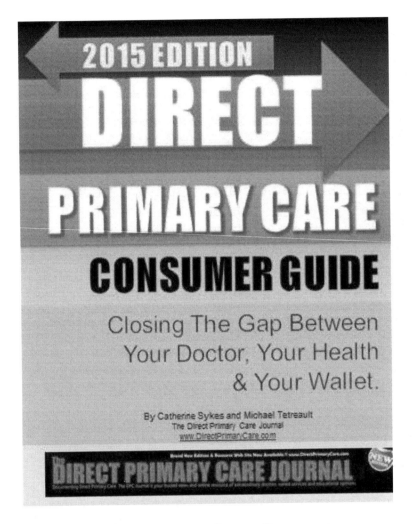

Available At:

When Patients Of Concierge Medical Care Were Asked To Weigh-In On Why They Choose Concierge Medical Care, They Said...

ConciergeMedicineToday.com and The Concierge Medicine Research Collective © 2012

- 34% said price was the main reason they chose concierge medical care.
- 29% said insurance compatibility was the main reason they chose concierge medical care.
- 17% said Medicare acceptance/participation was the main reason they chose concierge medical care.
- 6% said more time with my doctor was the main reason they chose concierge medical care.
- 6% said less office staff to deal with was the main reason they chose concierge medical care.
- 2% said limited/no waiting was the main reason they chose concierge medical care.
- 6% indicated a variety of other reasons not included in the list above.

How Does DPC and Concierge Medicine work with High Deductible Health Plans and Health Savings Accounts (HSAs)?

HSAs complement DPC and Concierge Medicine and clinics in a variety of ways.

Sue, who works inside a Concierge Medicine clinic in Washington State asks, "Many of our Patients are asking about HSAs and if they can use those funds to pay for the monthly fee associated with the practice. We charge a monthly fee and do not bill insurance, nor can the Patient submit for reimbursement. The fee covers any and all expenses in the office. Can you give me some information or advice to pass on to our Patients?"

Roy Ramthun a HSA expert based in Washington, DC, says "The IRS does not generally consider the monthly payment a 'qualified medical expense.' However, we do believe that they will accept reimbursements from an HSA for actual services provided by your practice physicians if you can produce something for the Patient that they can use to document the services they received (including any procedure/treatment codes), the date they were provided (and by whom), and the amount you would charge the Patient for the services provided. I know your practice is not set up that way, but the Patient needs something that tells them the fair market value of the services they received for tax-free reimbursement from their HSA."

The high deductible coverage from the HSA provides catastrophic protection against large or unexpected medical bills. The DPC or Concierge Medicine relationship with your physician will take care of routine medical needs and preventive care. The money saved on premiums for a HSA-qualified plan can help one fund a HSA account and/or pay for annual Concierge Medicine practice fees.

In addition, the HSA account can be used to reimburse the Doctor part of the cost of their Concierge Medical Services. While a Patient cannot pay an entire annual DPC or Concierge

Medicine practice fee with HSA funds without penalty. Patients can use a HSA funds tax-free to pay for individual medical services that are received from a Concierge Physician. This requires the physician to generate a "fee-for-service" bill indicating the type of medical care delivered (with appropriate codes) and the amount the Physician would normally charge for those services. This is the amount a Patient can withdraw tax-free from a HSA account. Over time, these withdrawals can help reimburse the annual cost of concierge medical services. Remember, reimbursement is not required if the Patient would prefer to save the money for future needs.

"DPC can complement High Deductible Health Plans (HDHPs), taking care of the primary care component of health care," adds Dr. Qamar. "HDHPs, or major medical plans, can take care of catastrophes. This combination can result in significant savings overall. Health Savings Accounts (HSAs), when structured properly with DPC plans, can also be used. The key is working with a DPC company, like MedLion, that has unquestionable legal and insurance knowledge."

What Is The Point Where DPC And Concierge Medicine Ends And Insured Care Begins?

Patients who are under the care of a Concierge Medicine physician or DPC doctor are encouraged to have insurance through a PPO, Medicare or a major medical plan. This allows for coverage of services provided outside of the doctor's office, such as catastrophic accidents, labs, radiology studies, specialty care and hospitalization. Concierge Medicine and care administered under the practice of a DPC clinic or physician are not considered pre-paid medical care. It is also important to recognize that Concierge Medicine or a fee paid to a DPC clinic or doctor is not considered a type of insurance coverage, company or product. Payment to these types of doctors or clinics in the form of a retainer or membership fee entitles Patients to office-based services and telephone conferences as needed, but not hospitalization or care provided by specialists.

Dr. Qamar says, "In paying directly for care, the line is drawn when the consumer can no longer afford to pay for services, usually after basic primary care services. DPC can offer affordable provider visits, labs, imaging, and medicine. Care beyond primary care is where insurance comes in handy. Examples are hospitalizations, surgical procedures, and specialist care."

We have found that approximately 80% of Concierge Doctors' offices participate in Medicare or various PPO insurance plans. Medicare and private insurances do not cover the annual fee. This is a completely separate fee that is paid directly to the doctor or doctor's office in return for enhanced access and other related services. Out-of-office charges and services provided by specialists and hospitalization expenses are billed directly to the Patient's insurance company or Medicare. Many Concierge Doctors' offices will bill Patients' insurance company or Medicare for services outside of the service contract agreed to between the Physician and the Patient.

While many news reports were focused on the problems with healthcare.gov and the online health marketplaces launched in October 2013, a growing number of people have found another option through participation in DPC and Concierge Medicine practices.

"I'm a self-pay Patient." says Eric in Millersport, OH. "Apparently, the modern health care business model no longer knows what to do with people like me. I'm a person, not a set of billing codes. I shouldn't have to deal with 4 separate bills from one trip to the Doctor. I shouldn't have to jump through hoops to find out what my lab work is going to cost just so that I can pay for it on the same day I get the work done. My medical care should be between me and my doctor. I see no reason why there need to be a half dozen corporate bureaucrats involved. I think you get the drift."

Initially such "highly cost medicine" came at a very high price, ranging upwards of $5,000 to $10,000 per Patient per year. Today, over 63% of the fees touted by DPC or Concierge Medicine doctors cost Patients less than $135 per month, according to *Concierge Medicine Today*.

Now offered by over approximately 12,000 physicians throughout the U.S. and growing, finding a physician in your local area will be important.

We have learned that over 80% of Concierge Medicine clinics still accept or participate in insurance (i.e. HMO, PPO, Medicare, Etc.). One hundred percent of both DPC and concierge medical care provided by a clinic or physician does not include specialty or hospital care. These types of practices often recommend that their members obtain a high-deductible wraparound policy to cover emergencies and catastrophic events.

Efforts are underway to combine changes in plan design with the DPC purchasing methodology. To date, two insurance carriers have tailored offerings to DPC-based Patients — Cigna and Associated Mutual. Cigna has pared its "Level Pay" program targeting self-insured employers with 50 to 250 employees and is offering this only to Qliance employer clients so far.

Erika Bliss, M.D., of Seattle, has been immersed in the DPC model since 2006. She is one of the founders of Qliance Medical Management. As president and CEO, she oversees a network of DPC clinics in the state that benefited from millions of dollars in capital investment from private business.

Bliss, a family physician who carves out 25 percent of her time for direct Patient care, said that the Qliance clinics had grabbed the attention of payers, purchasers and the government. "Large purchasers of health care (corporations) are saying 'This makes sense — you work hard on things that matter, not cranking out a bunch of visits and billing for them.'"

"Insurers recognize the potential for this model as well. Some are looking at insurance plans that work with DPC clinics to keep costs and premiums down," said Bliss.

Expedia, Inc., one of the world's leading online travel companies has partnered with Qliance, a leading healthcare organization operating a network of clinics that provide comprehensive primary care services, to open an onsite clinic at its Bellevue, Washington headquarters. Now, Expedia, Inc. employees and their dependents have easy access to primary health care services, including Saturday hours. The company hopes this effort will help prevent treatable symptoms from becoming chronic issues and encourage employees to use their sick time and medical benefits when needed. In just the first month of operation, employees and their dependents utilized nearly 300 office visits at the clinic.

"We are really pleased at how much use the clinic has received so far," said Connie Symes, Executive Vice President of Human Resources at Expedia, Inc. "It is great to see that the tools being provided are making health and well-being more convenient and accessible. As an employer, we spend a great deal of time attracting the best and brightest talent and we are equally focused on helping them be active and engaged employees of Expedia, Inc. We have a vested stake in the vitality of our workforce, and so we really cannot afford *not* to make preventative care a top priority for our employees."

Sharon, an Office Administrator at a DPC Clinic in Maryland asks "Can DPC fees be paid from an HSA?"

Roy Ramthun, a HSA expert based in Washington, DC, "No this has never been clarified. Advise Patients they cannot deduct or pay their annual fees with HSA dollars or other similar accounts. They should be able to reimburse fees for individual services if the doctor can produce a fee-for-service bill."

Associated Mutual has stated it is offering a wraparound policy but has not announced details yet. Physician Care Direct is working with DPC practices and networks, as well as multiple carriers, to facilitate wider adoption of the DPC model. They expect the combined cost of the DPC wraparound policy and DPC fees to be less than a standard health insurance plan.

Industry sources also tell us that a DPC clause was written into the Affordable Care Act (ACA) allowing retainer practices to be included in the proposed insurance exchanges, with the caveat that these practices be paired with a wraparound insurance policy covering services outside of primary care. According to a 2013 report by the California HealthCare Foundation, *It is the only non-insurance offering to be authorized in the insurance exchanges slated to begin in 2014; however, there is no requirement that DPCs be included.*

Concierge Medicine Offers Deeply Discounted Services To Patients

DPC doctors and Concierge Medicine physicians both help keep costs for Patients by avoiding unnecessary referrals and through referring to ancillary and imaging services willing to offer significant discounts.

How deep?

Dr. Robert Nelson of MyDoc in the Atlanta metro area, a DPC doctor, states "If you walk into a Quest or Lab Corp facility the cash price for a routine blood chemistry panel (CMP) will be $62.58 and $46, respectively. I can offer the same exact lab test to my Patients for $15, which covers my costs and the time related to clinical follow up as well. This shows the power of free-market leverage when you get out from under the third-party payment model. The good news is that these direct fees paid to DPC physicians or discount labs can still be applied towards deductibles and always go towards total out-of-pocket expenses for the year."

CNNMoney reports "By cutting out the middleman, [one doctor] said he can get a cholesterol test done for $3, versus the $90 the lab company he works with once billed to insurance carriers. An MRI can be had for $400, compared to a typical billed rate of $2,000 or more."

Interestingly, this is all happening at a time when the rise of health care costs has gone into pause.

"I have noticed that any Patient that comes in as a "cash pay" will always pay less than what a hospital or imaging center is billing the insurance for the same test. Also, remember, that some tests ordered are not typically covered by insurance (like a coronary CT) so, cash prices are extraordinarily important for these scenarios," says Dr. Tiffany Sizemore-Ruiz, a Concierge Doctor in the Miami/Fort Lauderdale Area.

The actual cost of medical care fell for first time since Gerald R. Ford was president of the United States.

"I can get much cheaper prices for my Patients. My PSA's are $30.00 and Lipids $15.00 ... and that is with a mark-up. General Health Screens (CBC, Thyroid, Liver Kidney and glucose tests) are $35 at my office. Next door at the lab, GHS SOT is greater than $200 and Lipids are higher than $100," says Dr. Tiffany Sizemore-Ruiz.

What Is Behind The Slowdown In Health Care Spending?

Clark Howard writes, 'First, employers are switching to high deductible health plans where you are responsible for so many thousands of dollars upfront before the company picks up the tab. When that happens, you start to treat health care like a consumer and become more cost conscious. Second, generic drugs are on the rise, which keeps the cost of health care down.'

Bob Adelmann wrote in *The New American*, 'Naturally the insurance industry isn't too happy about it, but at present there is little they can do. For the moment, "concierge" medicine and its more modest iteration, "direct pay" medicine, is increasingly being seen by Patients and doctors alike as a way out of the maze of medical practice requirements caused by government intervention in what used to be a simple transaction: a private matter between a doctor and his Patient.'

"Overall, concierge patients skew upper middle class, with typical household earnings between $125,000 and $250,000 a year, according to Michael Tetreault, Editor-in-Chief of Concierge Medicine Today, which covers the industry. They also tend to be Baby Boomers, generally in their 50s to 80s, according to doctors interviewed.
-CNN Money Interview, December 23, 2014

"We do not drift in good directions.
We discipline and prioritize ourselves there."

-Andy Stanley

A Concierge Doctor Does Not Have To Look At A Medical Chart To Know Your Name.

When was the last time your doctor inspired you to do the right thing for your health or the health of your family? When was the last time your doctor didn't have to look at your medical file or chart to know your name? These are compelling questions that cause Patients to think.

In the new world of medicine, medical homes, DPC and Concierge Medicine practices are delivering some very big results. The health care providers and the medical offices they operate are becoming so successful in today's over-crowded marketplace because of the simplicity of its delivery. The marketplace is ready for this type of healthcare delivery model and people are looking for alternatives to expensive health insurance. Not to mention, there is a huge uninsured population in America that cannot afford typical health insurance – concierge medical care is perfect for them at approximately $135 per month for more than sixty percent of the doctors' fees out there right now.

A new generation of people are lining up at doctor's offices across the U.S. and abroad to experience old-fashioned healthcare with a modern, relational twist. The idea of a doctor who sees them without delay, returns phone calls promptly, sends us emails, video chats and receives texts is completely foreign. Doctors like this, work in medical offices across the country and are now offering their Patients affordable access and personal attention when insurance is a hassle and time is tight.

So, what exactly is making these concierge medical homes attractive, affordable and inviting to everyone? It is summed up in five words: Price; Compatibility; Relationship; Technology; and Accessibility.

In Thomas Goetz's article *"How To Spot The Future"* published in April 2012 edition of *WIRED*, he outlined seven principles that underlie many of our contemporary innovations. He writes ... 'Odds are that any idea we deem potentially transformative, any trend we think has legs, draws on one or more of these core principles. They have played a major part in creating the world we see today. And they'll be the forces behind the world we'll be living in tomorrow ... First, look for cross-pollinators. It is no secret that the best ideas—the ones with the most impact and longevity—are transferable; an innovation in one industry can be exported to transform another. But even more resonant are those ideas that are cross-disciplinary not just in their application but in their origin.'

The vitality we see in today's Concierge Medicine marketplace resulted from the recognition that long wait times, overburdened physicians and insurance hassles aren't exclusive to the practice of medicine. In the past two decades, doctors have gone from completing six-hours of paperwork in order to provide a Patient with a $4 prescription to routinely emailing, phoning or texting their Patients, using Skype visit and iPhone cameras to dispatch medical advice. These doctors have opened up successful practices and there — eagerly incorporating ideas like: home visits; free medical advice; treatment of out-of-town family members; cloud-based medical records accessible and updatable anywhere; and prescription writing methods into their medical bag. These add tremendous benefit to Patients for a fraction of the cost that doctors' appointments, insurance fees and hospital visits would cost an individual.

Our hope is that by the time you are done reading this book, you will talk about Concierge Medicine being "the oldest, new form of medicine." We also hope that you will understand and share this information with your family and friends and tell them that Concierge Medicine is one of the oldest, proven, free-market healthcare delivery solutions available to anyone at a fraction of the cost of what the media has told you. These doctors are trying to reframe the identity of their practice and eventually the medical industry. And as Goetz says, ... 'that is testimony to a wave of cross-pollination.'

If you'd like to read Goetz's entire WIRED article, visit: http://www.wired.com/business/2012/04/ff_spotfuture/all/.

For Patients, the much-touted benefit of Concierge Medicine is that the doctor has more time and can provide them greater access. Concierge Doctors have 80% to 90% fewer Patients, so they have time to do things that other physicians simply cannot.

-Concierge Medicine Today, November 2013

Concierge Doctors are on the forefront of modern business and innovation. Like many modern medical practices across America, Concierge Medicine, DPC clinics and retail medicine offices are actually starting to list their prices to Patients before they require them to make a purchase.

Until recently, primary care and most health care practices were one of the only businesses in America that rarely listed how much they charged for services and products. The eventual evolution of concierge healthcare business models changed all of that. When the 2008 election and 2008 recession came ... the world of healthcare in America changed as we know it, forever. People started paying more attention to their credit card statements, health insurance claims, hospital bills and prescription drug costs.

Now with the emergence and passing of a sweeping federal statute, the Patient Protection and Affordable Care Act (PPACA), commonly called Obamacare has come into play. It raises a lot of questions for Doctors and Patients today who are trying to be served by a heavily regulated, insurance-based American model of healthcare that is not paying the doctors enough to stay in practice. It certainly isn't treating the Patients with the time and care everyone deserves. Not to mention, Doctors and Patients coping with the reality of Medicare benefit cuts and lower reimbursements are causing many people [and doctors] to search for an alternative ... those alternatives include Concierge Medicine and DPC business models.

Rx Compliance Among Concierge Medicine Patients

The online and offline chatter about the overall health benefits for a Patient inside a concierge medical practice has been well documented by bloggers, the media and even physician associations over past years. There is still quite a bit of mystery surrounding this topic but one recent interview and discussion between our Editors and a **Fortune 50 Drug Corporation** reveals some fascinating insight. According to a recent interview with an Executive at the company, Patients who have a concierge physician are far less reliant on prescription medications than those Patients at a traditional primary care or family practice. In some cases, Concierge Physicians can reduce the total amount of medication their Patients take by 50-95%, this according to surveys obtained from concierge/direct care physicians operating in the concierge medical movement across the U.S.

What does this mean for the drug companies promoting drugs and educating physicians about certain medications to concierge physicians? Our source continued to say that this drop in the use of prescription medication was immediately noticed by high-level executives within the company and caused a slight shift in the sales strategy among the sales reps in the field. That strategic thinking and sales strategy reduced the amount of time anyone prescription sales rep spends calling on Concierge Medical or DPC practices, compared to a more traditional, insurance based medical practice.

There may however be a side to this story that is not so familiar to the drug manufacturers. Concierge Medicine practices may actually help to improve medication compliance, which is the Patient's consistency in taking prescribed medications over time . In 2011, preliminary research was conducted by *The Concierge Medicine Research Collective* and *Concierge Medicine Today*. They found that among concierge physicians across the U.S., when physicians were asked to ' grade their concierge medical Patients' on medication compliance, ' 96.3% of the doctors indicated that 75% of their Patients comply with prescription regimens all or most of the time.

When compared to traditional medical practices or insurance/MCO based medical practices, concierge medical doctors have more time to research the drugs they prescribe (up to 4 hours per day in some cases according to *Concierge Medicine Today* internal analysis) and these physicians are able to spend more time explaining the prescription usage, history and benefits to Patients. In fact, in the majority of office visits conducted inside concierge physician practices in 2010, a single office visit with a concierge physician can last as little as 45 minutes and as long as 3 hours in some cases. Medication compliance is a Patient health issue, since not taking medication may slow or prevent recovery, or even worsen the Patient's condition. However, poor compliance is also a topic that drug manufacturers pay attention to, since it means poor sales of prescriptions and refills as well.

A 2005 Harris Interactive report indicates that roughly half of all prescriptions for drugs meant to be taken on an ongoing basis are either not completed or are never filled in the first place. Surveys conducted from January 2010 to present among Concierge Physicians by *Concierge Medicine Today* indicate that 'the most common types of phone calls Concierge Physicians receive from their Patients' were prescription drug renewal requests. These accounted for 35% of all calls while the other most common being Cold/Flu Symptoms (20%) and Back pain 15%.

When Concierge Physicians were asked 'Do you see a difference in how well concierge Patients follow through and/or comply with taking prescription medications, as opposed to Patients you have treated in traditional practice?' the following results were found:

- 67% - of respondents polled indicated that Yes! A Significant Difference;
- 28% - Some, but not a big difference; and
- 6% - No difference at all.

When these same Concierge Doctors were asked 'If you have noticed your concierge Patients do better when taking their Rx meds, what do you think accounts for this change?' we found the following results:

- 38% - I follow up personally to ask about medication use and side effects, and to encourage compliance.
- 28% - I spend more time explaining the importance of medication compliance.
- 28% - The Patient has more confidence in my recommendations and will follow them.
- 7% - Other.

Concierge Physicians may indeed take a more conservative approach to prescribing multiple medications, but their high level of attention to Patient care may at the same time promote greater medication compliance. Is one to presume that Patients who have a Concierge Physician develop closer relationships with their doctors and therefore respond more positively to medical advice? That could be the case. The hallmark of concierge medical care is the doctors more personalized approach to treating individual Patients, which in turn allows more time to research appropriate treatment alternatives and spend more time counseling and following up with Patients. As the drug company executive noted, one outcome of concierge care is fewer prescriptions. However, the high proportion of prescription requests suggests Concierge Medicine Patients may also exhibit higher levels of medication compliance. This is a topic we will explore further in the future.

What Is The Annual Income Of The Typical Concierge Medical Patient In 2011?
© 2013, The Concierge Medicine Research Collective

- 34% – earn less than $100,000 each year and regularly use concierge medical care
- 39% – earn between $100k-200k per year and regularly use concierge medical care
- 14% – earn between $200k-$300k per year and regularly use concierge medical care
- 5% – earn between $300k-$400k per year and regularly use concierge medical care
- 3% – earn between $400k-$500k per year and regularly use concierge medical care
- 2% – earn between $500k-$600k per year and regularly use concierge medical care
- 1% – earn between $600k-$700k per year and regularly use concierge medical care
- 2% – earn between $700k and above per year and regularly use concierge medical care

We recently submitted this data to a prominent financial magazine and told them that 'Utilizing a blended rate based upon national averages for current fees charged for concierge medical care, an estimated 9,285,714,286 people could be provided concierge medical care with the 13 trillion dollar debt. Carrying this out 928,571,429 people could be provided this care for 10 years. These figures are based upon information obtained through average pricing surveys conducted from 2009-2010 by *Concierge Medicine Today (CMT)*.'

Be sure that on your web site you have pictures of the outside of your office. You'd be surprised how many times Patients get lost and drive right by a doctor's office. The more information you can give them to help relieve the stress of visiting the doctor's office, the better. It is also helpful to have nice pictures of your staff also. Make your Patients feel as comfortable as possible.

-Bestselling Book, The Marketing MD, © 2014

"Some doctors would say this is easy, especially the successful ones," says Matthew Priddy, MD, who operates in a thriving concierge medicine practice based in Indianapolis, IN. "But there are also doctors who failed, gave up, and went back and worked for hospitals. Those folks are out there too, and they would probably tell you that it's impossible. It can be a little bit of a selection bias when you talk to the doctors who are oft-quoted in the media or who are involved in national organizations. But that is more the exception than the norm."

Chapter 6 –
Are We There Yet?
Generating Buzz & Growing Your Medical Practice.

Key Performance Indicators (KPIs) And Your Success

Key Performance Indicators (KPI), also known as Key Success Indicators (KSI), help a concierge medical practice define and measure progress toward organizational goals (Source: About.com). Once a private practice has analyzed its mission, identified all its audience, and defined its goals, it needs a way to measure progress toward those goals. Key Performance/Success Indicators are those measurements.

Many aspects of your concierge medical practice are measurable. In selecting your KPIs, limiting them to topics that are essential to reaching your quarterly and annual goals is very important. Keeping the number of KPIs you follow modest enough to keep your staff's attention focused on achieving those same KPIs is also crucial. Let's take a look at a few here.

Patient Indicators

There are a variety of ways to measure Patient satisfaction. Verbal questions with later documented notes, Patient feedback forms, social media surveys, social media comments and recommendations recorded on your Practice Facebook or Google+ Business Page — and other such methods are great ways to quantify and examine Patient satisfaction. We might think that after a month or two of operating that everything is going smoothly, but there are usually small things that Patients pick up on and can suggest that you (or in many cases, your staff) could do better. Documenting and examining these KPIs quarterly or even annually at the very least will help you make small, and sometimes critical, improvements.

The most successful concierge medical practices are the ones that communicate regularly with the majority (if not all) of their Patients on a routine basis that makes their Patients feel like the Doctor is reaching out and maintaining a connection. It does not have to be face-to-face either. Many times, a simple text, Skype visit or phone call will suffice.

However, if your front-office employees are not specifically asking each Patient whether They have visited your practice in the past and **'is there anything else we can do to improve your next visit?'** ... this KPI can be difficult to track and start to increase annual Patient attrition. One example we can all relate to is a recent trip to the grocery store. We have all heard a check-out counter employee ask us 'did you find everything you were looking for today?' While this type of service may seem inconsequential, it still means something in the service industry. Think about what questions you'd like to be asked and ask your employees to do the same. You will probably be surprised at the responses.

Five (5) Staff Interactions At Your Concierge Medical Practice That Should Never Happen

The lobby of your medical practice and reception area says more to your Patients than anywhere else in your practice. If it is furnished well, tidy and the staff working in this area are well-trained, helpful, smiling and friendly, this can be a good thing. But if not, it can be a very bad thing.

Each day, you want Patients to walk into your practice, not judge it. So, make sure you do the following things:

Make Patients feel unwelcome. Patients at your practice should always feel welcome. That means greeting each Patient as they arrive with a smile (even if your staff does not feel like it) and friendliness. Go out of your way to be courteous at all times. If you have a service window in your lobby area, remember that your staff represents you and the demeanor of your practice, so they have to be smiling and friendly at all times.

Do Not Be Too Casual. The flip side of not being friendly enough is being a bit too friendly. Your service window staff should never interrupt a conversation. No matter how casual the atmosphere around your practice is, your staff must always be professional. Even if someone is in pain, aggravated or disruptive, they deserve to be treated with kindness and respect.

Do Not Hide Things. Nothing is worse than finding out you owe money from a previous visit, you owe more than a co-pay (if applicable in your practice), or your doctor is on vacation and you will be seeing a colleague. According to Concierge Medicine Today polls, these are the most common complaints among Patients inside a Concierge Medicine office. Service window staff should not lie to Patients, deceive them, or be anything other than honest. Is there a delay? Tell the Patients as soon as possible. Is there an upcharge for a certain test that was performed? Make sure to mention it. Always let Patients know before they leave of any increase in pricing of your services and when the practice is going to be closed during upcoming holidays.

Do Not Argue With Patients. This might seem obvious, but it is important. The phrase, *"The customer is always right"* is a cliché for a reason! When a Patient complains, employees should do their best to listen and help. Try to diffuse the situation by understanding and validating their feelings. You should try to fix a problem when possible, or refer the Patient to the Doctor or Office Manager if there is nothing certain staff can do. Never, ever fight with Patients or dispute their complaints, even if they are wrong. If it is something they are arguing with you about in the lobby, take the conversation to another part of the practice to discuss it. Nothing makes your practice look worse than bad word of mouth, arguing or gossip in front of current Patients.

Do Not Make The Patient Feel Rushed. This is Concierge Medicine. There should not be a rush! Did you know that more Patients leave a Concierge Medicine practice because they were over-promised and underserved? That is right. If you promise no-wait appointments, no rushed visits, deliver on your promises. When Patients come to your practice, it is for relief and peace of mind. What they do not want is to feel rushed and pushed out of the office so the next Patient can be served. Isn't that why you got into this practice in the first place? No matter how crazy the office gets or how many people are waiting on a busy day, make sure Patients feel as relaxed and comfortable as possible.

Staff Indicators

Did you realize that a significant number of Patients leave their concierge practice each year because of ill-tempered or rude personnel employed by the doctor's office? That is right. Often the staff member has been employed for a number of years and the doctor believes they are indispensable. The following staff performance indicators will help you keep track of data so you can monitor how well your employees are impacting the success of your practice. Pay attention to the total labor cost indicator, especially if you are a relatively new Concierge Medicine medical practice owner (less than 5 years), because it centers on how your staff impacts your renewals and Patient volume.

Total labor cost: Total labor cost is one of the largest expenses you will incur as a medical office owner. In a lot of Concierge Medicine medical practice office settings, approximately 38% of the practices' annual expenditures are paid to employees and part-time staff. Hence, the reason you must consistently keep track of this. According to an article in the *Houston Chronicle*, labor cost should range on average from 25 to 35 percent of your total expenses. Total labor cost includes salary or hourly wages, benefits, insurance, retirement, and bonuses that you pay to yourself and your employees.

Labor hours: How many hours do your employees work during a certain time frame? You should compare these hours against your sales to measure the productivity of your staff.

Turnover: Count the positions you employ, and then divide this number by the number of people you have employed during a certain period of time. For example, if you have two staff positions and you have employed six people in the last year, your staff turnover is 1/3 or 30 percent.

Patient Attrition: How many Patients DO NOT renew their membership annually? Survey these Patients to determine their reasons. If is often advisable to have an outside or objective party conduct the survey as a Patient may be reticent to reveal dissatisfaction with the staff or doctors service directly to a staff member or to the doctor directly. We ask routinely hundreds of concierge medical doctors 'what is your largest annual expense?' Our sources from tell us that Concierge Medicine doctors' offices spend about 38% of their annual income on Staff/employees followed closely by Leased Office Space/Mortgage at 24%. In a close third, Malpractice Insurance at 19% and equipment at 5% and rising.

"It is high time that the ideal of success
should be replaced by the ideal of service."

~Albert Einstein

Marketing and Advertising Indicators

This list of indicators is more important to Concierge Medical and DPC practice owners who actually spend money on marketing. A large majority of doctors do. Most Concierge Doctors spend as little as 5% on marketing and advertising each year where some doctors choose to spend more – surveys tell us as much as 14% of their annual income. Many new concierge medical practice owners start up without putting any funding into this area, and thus do not need to track this data. While it can be very difficult to grow a private-pay practice in a difficult economy, many Concierge Medicine doctors are thriving … increasing their annual revenue each year in the first five years from $100K per year to $400,000 or more per year.

We have been asking doctors important questions for a very long time. One of those questions is 'How long does it take to recruit or persuade a new Patient to become a Patient in your practice?' Another one is 'What form of marketing is most productive when trying to attract new Patients to your practice?' The answers to these questions are critical for your success and give you an advantage others never had.

How Long Does It Take To Recruit Or Persuade 'One' New Patient To Become A Patient In Your Practice?
© 2013, The Concierge Medicine Research Collective

- 49% – Four or more months
- 23% – Three to four months
- 4% – One to two months
- 13% – Two to four weeks
- 11% – One to two weeks

What form of marketing is most productive when trying to attract new Patients to your practice?
© 2013, The Concierge Medicine Research Collective

- 16% – Hire a Marketing/PR Firm
- 14% – Letter with Brochure
- 13% – Word of Mouth Referral

With a natural attrition rate of roughly 10% (according to our industry analyses), is only one of the following ways listed above enough to sustain a practice year after year? A doctor will know when they consistently track and measure the following KPIs in this category:

- Marketing and public relations (PR) costs
- Response rates
- Sales inquiry conversion rate
- Press mentions

If you ask Patients for e-mail addresses in order to provide them
with special offers or for Patient referral bonuses — this type of marketing costs you
considerably less than having to advertise and market for a new Patient in your local newspaper
or networking event.

~Book, Branding Concierge Medicine, © 2011

Sales and Service Indicators

These indicators center on your bottom line. Your sales and service costs will determine whether your concierge medical practice is succeeding financially.

Service cost percentage: How much do you spend per Patient to make sure your practice is 'servicing' your Patient to the level they'd like? This may include equipment expenditures, magazine subscriptions, beverage delivery, television/cable costs, vitamins, recipe cards, etc. Think of these as the non-medical and non-health related add-ons that Patients know make your practice different from other doctors' offices in the area. These services are not part of your square footage fee in your lease agreement or mortgage.

You usually calculate these costs as a percentage of your total business expense. You measure it by adding your purchases for the week and comparing those figures to your weekly sales. Depending on the type of services you provide to your Patients, this number can range from 5 to 15 percent. (*Note:* Doctors' offices that choose the route of operating a franchised practice model will have a lower service cost potentially due to the buying power and cost control systems the franchisor can bring or limitation of services they accept inside a new franchised practice.)

Weekly sales: This number is one of the standard sales-related numbers that every doctor's office should look at. As you may expect, weekly sales can vary widely from one practice to the next. The key number to look at is any change you find from week to week and how it compares to previous years.

Sales per head: One of the most used performance indicators is sales per head, which you calculate by dividing your total sales by the number of Patients you serve. To do this, you must make sure your point-of-sale system or your employees and staff are properly accounting for the number of Patients each sale covers. You can calculate your sales per head at different times or shifts throughout the day, week, month or quarter. For a more detailed understanding of this metric, you can track your sales per head each week or month to look for reasons for positive or negative trends. For example, your sales per head may trend downward when you run discounted product-related (i.e. add-on) specials.

Best (and worst) selling items: Check the weekly sales from your receipts or point-of-sale system to help you determine which services from your menu items are either consistently selling out or simply taking up space on your menu board.

"We do all the membership admin in house and do not lose profits. I much prefer it this way and so do the Patients. I have 350 Patients, and about to hire a PA. We have two local employers who would like us to manage their 40 employees each, and possibly families, since they will be changing their insurance plans due to Obamacare. I am looking at sort of a hybrid private member/corporate member structure, which I think will be a good balance. We can then offer onsite services for their employees without increasing our overhead or need for space. The possibilities are endless..."

-Dr. Jennifer Chilek
Montgomery, TX | Stone Creek Family Medicine

PR, Marketing and Branding Concierge Medicine

16 Ways To Update Your Concierge or DPC Practice Business Plan For Better Results

One thing almost all Concierge, DPC and private-pay medical practice owners around the U.S. need is more Patients. Have you ever wondered how proper business planning can help you find new Patients for your new practice model? The key for any physician/business owner is to take a step back from your daily routine and reconsider your strategy. Additionally, what strategies have impacted Patient volume at your practice the most in the past six or even twelve months? While you were busy building your practice, your local market or your Patient-base may have changed slightly. Economics sure have shifted recently in almost every small town and suburb. How has your practice responded to Patients watching their bottom-line even more closely than before? You can sometimes identify these changes by asking other physicians, searching online or joining a social media group to give yourself some new angles.

After all this, your goal should be to redevelop your concierge/private practice business plan by adding new marketing/sales initiatives to your practice. Each strategy should involve specific responsibilities that can be assigned to specific people within your practice — with deadlines, start dates and anticipated budgetary costs.

We have put together a few proven strategies that should set you on a path to finding new Patients for your modern medical home and hopefully to higher annual revenue as well:

STRATEGY # 1 —

Follow A Strategic Marketing Plan Because It Works.

We have talked to countless Concierge and DPC doctors over the years and spoken with many at conferences and seminars. They seem to always say the same thing, 'Traditional advertising mediums just do not get it done and I do not have the money to spend on marketing.' My response is usually, where are you spending your money? They reply, 'I do not know. I did a postcard and pay-per-click on Google for a couple of months. Neither worked very well.'

Growing a medical practice takes money, maybe not that much ... but typically, successful [primary care, specialty and family] medical practices across the U.S. that we have seen and worked with budget between 3% to 8% of their annual budget. But to the un-learned medical professionals, when we think about marketing, we think it is going to cost a lot of money to find out what is going to stick to the wall and actually work.

The best way to overcome this unrest in your mind and wallet is to create a written plan. Tell your dollars where they are going to be spent on paper, on purpose. Wouldn't you feel more comfortable knowing exactly where every dollar is going before you spent them?

The average family out-of-pocket expenditures in 2013 now exceed $20,000 per year. The growth of retail medicine, DPC, urgent care, Concierge Medicine and nurse-staffed wellness clinics are increasing provider choice – allowing Patients more affordable and faster options for a Patient. By late 2014, 80 million lives should have been buying their own health insurance, thereby increasing health plan choices for millions of prospective Patients.

Proper, well-thought out, methodical and planned marketing plans show you where you will spend your money. It is up to you to decide where you will actually spend these dollars. That in itself takes some time and research.

The promotion of your private-pay, DPC or Concierge Medical practice requires personal interaction with current and prospective Patients to create interest in your services, staff and practice. Since "prospective Patients" include current Patients that may become repeat visitors, promotion can happen inside as well as outside of the practice.

Try some of these tactics to promote your Concierge Medical or DPC practice:

STRATEGY # 2 —

Review your pricing.

Price is the most powerful marketing message you have. What is most important isn't the high or low of it, but how it matches your strategy. When *Concierge Medicine Today* asked current Patients of Concierge Medicine medical practice, 'what is the most common objection you have that influences your decision when choosing a private, Concierge Doctor is ...' 34% said price is biggest concern/objection they have, followed closely by insurance compatibility at 29%.

Some Concierge Medical practices are built around visible, low-priced services aimed to bring people up to their service window and generate higher unit sales. Others offer more personal services and sprinkle in more relational ingredients into their business plan aimed at meeting a need at a higher price and communicating a message routinely to Patients that keeps them coming back for more assistance. A problem with frequent low pricing is that your concierge/private medical practice may wind up losing Patients who assume your stable of services are not keeping pace with their needs.

Should you decide to revise your pricing, make sure you reflect that in your sales forecast, research your competitors, analyze your marketplace and insert it appropriately into your overall marketing messages when necessary. While you may think the marketplace can bear a higher retainer/annual fee for your service, be cautious and analyze thoroughly before taking action steps. A knowledgeable marketing consultant can assist you with these types of analyses. At CMT, we have a list of Endorsed Local Providers that we can refer you to and help you make some of these decisions.

STRATEGY # 3 —

Review your marketing messages.

That means both the core content of your message, and how you are delivering it. In all direct-pay models, Patients communicate in various ways. Some prefer SMS Text, some email, some face-to-face and some over the phone. Most recently, we have seen 'THANK YOU' NOTES coming back into the marketing mix – whereby doctors and their staff are encouraged to write thank you notes to Patients for something they may have learned from them during a recent visit. It could be a new web site, a recipe or something else of practical value to you and your staff that communicates to your Patients, 'thank you for your visit, I listened to you and I appreciate you.' Most Patients use social media – particularly Facebook, and LinkedIn to spread the word about how sick they are or how ill their kids are and they had to take a day off from work. Social media is a new form of word-of-mouth advertising. It would behoove you and your practice to, at the very least, start spreading the word on social media networks about what your practice has to offer.

Whatever strategy you decide on, make sure you consider adding these ideas and others to your existing Concierge Medicine or DPC practice business plan. As often as possible, include measurement and tracking methods so you can tell if you have successfully implemented the new idea. Then follow-up and review actual results in the next six to twelve months. You can see what is going right and what isn't, and make the necessary adjustments to maximize the profits your modern medical practice home brings in.

Find the bad apple (if you have one that is) and either reposition them to employment in the practice where direct Patient interaction is not required or ask them to potentially move on to another place of employment. Every small medical practice, particularly in Concierge Medicine or DPC has its own culture. It does not mean that all of your employees must think exactly the same way as you do. But by creating a set of shared beliefs, belief in your new business; pricing model; forecasted goals; and celebrated achievements internally causes everyone to have the same idea on how to accomplish their daily tasks, set priorities, make decisions, treat Patients, and treat each other. This is crucial to success.

-Catherine Sykes
Author, Speaker, Healthcare Strategist

Listing sites such as: Vitals.com; HealthyGrades.com; ZocDoc.com; GetListed.org; EverydayHealth.org; RateMDs.com; DrScore.com; Switchboard.com, Yahoo!, Bing, Google Local, YP.com, Kudzu.com and AngiesList.com allows searchers (i.e. prospective Patients) to narrow their search by categories of services and view past Patient reviews. It would make sense to take the time to monitor monthly these comments, tie your services to as many of these categories as possible so that your business appears in more instances when a person is searching. Most of these sites are free. Some require a subscription. Start using them today!

STRATEGY # 4 —

Micro Site and Online Reviews Matter.

See what is being said about you and your concierge medical or DPC practice inside the world of social media. Google, Bing and Yahoo! search can be very helpful with this. In the medical service and primary care marketplace, we both know that referrals are priority No. 1 when your prospective Patients are seeking out a physician to help them or their family. The online world has definitely broadened what a 'referral' means. If somebody sees enough positive reviews for a doctor, this helps people validate where they should go for their treatment and health care. The opposite also holds true. For many doctors and private concierge healthcare clinics, reputation management includes not just tracking positive news, but also guarding against the negative. These days, feedback on sites like "Yelp!," "Google+," "HealthyGrades" and "Yahoo! Local" can make a big difference to a doctor.

If you own a medical practice, there is no way around it: You need to follow general and industry-specific review sites. These are front-row seats to what your Patients and future Patients are saying about you ... specifically. That is incredibly valuable insight into Patient-perception and issues you may need to resolve, and even things you are doing very well.

STRATEGY # 5 —

Review and analyze regularly.

Finally, any promotional efforts you do must be remembered, recorded and analyzed. The goal here is to see what works, what does not work, and where your time and money are going. Often something doctors and office managers neglect for lack of time once the promotion is mailed out and the phone is ringing with results. Even things as simple as social media need to be reviewed quarterly. Are you using the right social platforms? Are you visiting them too infrequently to the point where you do not build up a regular following? Did you know that improvement in your search engine listing can take a minimum of 3 to 4 months before you start seeing your rankings increase. Do you come across as a spammer by constantly tweeting and sharing?

My advice is always look at what you do and how it is likely being perceived by the average consumer and future Patient.

"*The advertising aimed at them [seniors age 55+] is simply aimed at maintaining brand loyalty and establishing that the products [and services] they love are still good and still work and maybe are being improved. But you will not see advertising aimed at those people that is designed to get them to switch brands. The advertising aimed at 25-54 is all about that. And, by the way, not every advertising agency knows what it is doing.*"

~Rush Limbaugh, January 2014

STRATEGY # 6 —

Follow up personally with Patients.

You can do this both inside and outside of the practice. When currently practicing concierge physicians were asked, 'how much time do you spend of the phone each day with Patients?' the results were as follows:

- 2% – less than 1-10-minutes /day;
- 8% – less than 11-25-minutes /day;
- 14% – less than 26-35-minutes /day;
- 12% – 36-45 minutes /day;
- 10% – 61-90-minutes /day;
- 19% – 90-minutes – 3 hours per day.

After Patients complete their visit, it is never a bad idea for the doctor or Office Manager to speak with them directly, thanking them and asking if they were satisfied with everything. You can also follow up on customer service issues at this time as well. For example, if Patients fill out a comment card and leave negative comments, you could call them to apologize for their negative experience and offer to make up for it next time by fixing the problem and giving them a discount or something of 'unique value'.

STRATEGY # 7 —

Make friends using THANK YOU notes ....

It is old-fashioned but everyone loves to be thanked. The best part is, a person ALWAYS reads them and it goes a long way the next time you come up in conversation with friends, family, co-workers, etc.

STRATEGY # 8 —

Pitch to local companies.

You can speak personally with the human resources (HR) managers or appropriate personnel at any companies or factories that are in your local area to see if they are interested in setting up an appointment or having you host an educational (topic-focused) meeting or event at their company.

STRATEGY # 9 —

Contact local service organizations.

Ask the Chamber of Commerce or the convention center for a list of contact information for organizations, such as service organizations, unions, political organizations, etc. Call them and tell them about your practice. See if there are any opportunities for your practice to be presented. You may offer to write a column for their newsletter or do an educational session on a common healthcare concern. Be creative!

STRATEGY # 10 —

Keep magazines up-to-date.

If you are one of the rare private-pay, retainer, DPC or Concierge Doctors that still use a waiting room, there is nothing worse than outdated magazines on your table. Be sure to subscribe to the latest health and wellness magazines and be sure your staff tosses out anything older than last month.

STRATEGY # 11 —

Be friendly, not pushy.

Whenever you are talking to a prospective Patient, show excitement about what you have to offer, smile and be easy-going. If they are not very receptive of your new service offering, do not irritate them further.

STRATEGY # 12 —

Cross-Sell Services.

A basic and core principle that any marketing consultant worth their salt will tell you is ... you can sell new products/services to old clients and old products/services to new clients ... but never, under any circumstances try selling old products/services to old clients and new products/services to new clients. Hopefully that makes sense to you. Let me explain even further.

The quickest path to healthy bottom-line growth in a concierge/private medical practice is continuing to reinvent or reposition your services as unique so Patients will keep coming back to you for more help. One of the greatest challenges physicians like yourself face when starting these new Concierge Medicine medical homes is acquiring more new Patients.

When they have completed the transition and have an established Patient-base of around 300 Patients – the doctor starts to say 'I now need more Patients.' Well, this challenge puts you squarely in the box of taking a new service/business model to new, prospective Patients. We have learned from many doctors that for the majority (72%) of doctors trying to acquire new Patients into their practice, it is taking 3-4+ months to recruit one new Patient! The best story I have heard is the concierge/private physician that contacted her entire Patient base and reminded them all (via phone personal telephone call **from the doctor – not staff**) that they were approaching their prescription renewal and the doctor would like to see you — to review whether or not that medication was working, not working, needed to be adjusted and just in general, talk to the Patients about how things are going. This practice created a special promotion and cleared met some internal goals in the process.

How could something like that work for your practice? The story illustrates how Patients can be grateful for reminders, and be ready to say yes to improved relationship with their doctor and overall better quality health. Essentially, there are three parts to it: Determining what you can offer that relates to your Patients and practice offerings, how to turn these ideas into an event and how to get the message out to Patients.

When you come up with something, put it into the milestones of your business plan. Give it a start date, end date, and a person in charge. Estimate additional revenue so you will know, for next time, whether you underestimated or overestimated.

STRATEGY # 13 —

Use Facebook "Check-In" At Your Practice. Put A Stick On Your Front Door If You Have To!

Virtually every brand and business today has a Facebook Page. Unfortunately, medical practices are some of the last to adopt-a-page and jump into the social media-sphere. As most people are looking to fill idle time with smart phone usage, few medical practices have made their Facebook Business Page "local." All that practices have to do to make their Page "local" is to add an address to their Facebook Page settings.

Once an address is added, Facebook users will be able to check-in by either tagging their location in a post or by navigating to your page and clicking "check-in." Note that users must be within a certain radius before the "check-in" button will appear. tip; Make sure to change your Facebook Page "type" to "BRAND" or "LOCAL BUSINESS" in order to enable users to check-in. Otherwise, some Page types will not have an option to add an address.

STRATEGY # 14 —

Prepare A Tablet Strategy For Your Practice

More and more people are using tablets like the iPad to surf the web during business hours, waiting rooms, meetings and at home. Having free Wi-Fi in your office is a must! Searches among tablet users have increased exponentially in the past year and more PR agencies and small business promoters are encouraging business owners to stay updated in the latest technology trends by creating web sites, blogs and geo-targeted advertisements specific for tablets. This also includes the use of videos. So, while creating a tablet marketing strategy for your practice might seem like a time vacuum, it would be wise for you to consider talking to a web professional to help you prepare for the next phase in social connection.

Growing a medical practice takes money, maybe not that much ...
but typically, successful [primary care, specialty and family] medical practices across the U.S.
that we have seen and worked with budget between 3% to 8% of their annual budget. But to the un-
learned medical professionals, when we think about marketing, we think it is going to cost a lot of
money to find out what is going to stick to the wall and actually work.

~The Marketing MD, book, © 2013

STRATEGY # 15 —

Impulsive May Mean Broke

Since marketing budgets for small and medium practices are generally small, you cannot afford to over-spend, nor under-spend. You cannot afford to be impulsive either. In working with hundreds of small businesses over the years, we have found that the majority have wasted at least 70% of their marketing and advertising budgets because they really never learned, edited and mastered their marketing activities. They simply used the trial and error method and at times, focused on the urgent task when a supposedly 'great deal' came their way. This can torpedo any budget and waste a lot of money. Do not market your medical practice because you saw a competitor do something or a 'great deal' came your way.

In order to be successful in navigating a marketing map/plan, you must pay to play. Sponsoring a local middle-school soccer team and putting your name on the jerseys does not come free. Participating in a local health fair usually is accompanied by an entry fee. Mailing postcards to your Patients encouraging them to see your new office location isn't free. Knowing you must allow 3% to 8% of your annual budget each year for specific marketing tasks before we begin down the path of learning can be a difficult pill to swallow. But remember, there are no shortcuts. Very rarely will new Patients find you by accident. Steven Covey said "Most of us spend too much time on what is urgent and not enough time on what is important."

STRATEGY # 16 —

Holiday Marketing Seasonal Promotions

If it is the season to drape your signage and office lobby in greenery, twinkling lights, hang a "LIVE" Christmas wreath onto your door and get prepped for the onset of happy holiday Patients.

Busy Patients are out and about and rushing to get their last minute shopping done and more importantly, fill those last-minute prescriptions and forgotten office visits before the end of the year. That is where you come in. The holiday season is an ideal opportunity for you to soften the beaches in their minds that your medical practice is the best spot to stop and refuel and make sure your holiday season is a healthy one. It is also a time to draw their attention to refilling upcoming prescriptions, book January appointments, inform them about nutritional and healthy eating seminars you are planning to do in your office and tell them about a special holiday themed event or promotion you are running.

With an ounce of creativity, your holiday event or promotion can be as simple as dropping a holiday prescription reminder in the mail to each of your Patients or to tell them that a donation point for a local charity or that you are accepting canned goods for a holiday charity drive. The key is creating enough top of mind awareness to keep your medical practice on speed dial during a time when Patients are so easily distracted.

Here are three great ideas for driving foot traffic to your private-pay medical during the bustling holiday season.

1. Collect Canned Goods or Host a Charity Drive

Nothing shows goodwill during the holidays like giving to others. It is one of the easiest and most charitable efforts you can do each year and still involve your Patients. It is easy to advertise, easy to collect and easy to drop off donated items once the charity drive is over.

We recommend partnering with a locally based charitable organization for a holiday collection drive. Habitat For Humanity or the Habitat Home Store (if applicable) in your area might be looking for clothing, toiletry items, hammers, etc. Local churches, food banks and homeless shelters are always looking for partners to assist them in their community with the collection of canned goods, food, warm clothing, blankets and other items.

Ask your local area churches close to your practice about how you can help collect items and drop them off this holiday season. Then, send a list of these items to your Patients by email, in the office via a flyer, etc. Ask for support relating to your charity drive by promoting your practice and location through social media and email.

Besides doing something good for your community, if your Patients, Facebook fans or LinkedIn followers know that they can knock off to-do's on their list, fill their spouse's prescription, get a quick sore throat check-up and drop off a holiday donation, they are more likely to make a point of stopping by. Because space is an issue for medical practice owners, consider collecting smaller gifts such as pet toys for a local animal shelter or hygiene items for a homeless center and put the collection boxes, nicely decorated of course, and positioned in a prominent location where most of your Patients will see items being donated in your lobby or waiting area.

2. Hit the Mail

Holiday cards to your favorite Patients, drug and DME suppliers and physician supporters are a great way to encourage physician referrals towards your practice in the New Year. This not only creates a personal connection but it is also an opportunity you to slip in a note about your practice, special services you provide and about your charity drive throughout the season.

Handle the mailing yourself with an on-the-go compact mailing system or stamps.com so you can get your cards in the mail pronto. If you miss the post-Christmas mailing deadline, New Year's cards work just as well to remind your followers to stop in and book their next appointment.

3. Amp up Your Patient Testimonials, Online Reviews, Reputation and Social Media

There is nothing better than a great Patient testimonial. With the holidays upon them, people, especially your Patients, typically feel in a generous and giving mood. That being said, they'd probably enjoy writing a sentence or two about you, their experience with your practice and staff on one of the physician review web sites. Encourage them to do so!

4. You must have a Facebook Page. If not, get one. Now!

Facebook, Twitter, Instagram and Pinterest are thrifty and effective buzz-generating mediums for promoting just about anything, especially good word of mouth referrals. Create Facebook Events for each promotion and invite your friends. Post photos on Instagram of your holiday lights, your staff in elf hats, holiday treats, and happy Patients (with their permission of course). Create a Pinterest contest where customers can pin photos of their donation they brought into your office in order to qualify to win a free gift basket. The options are endless but bottom line, social media creates a visual online picture that your medical practice is the place to be during the holiday season.

Why Do Patients Leave A Concierge Physician?

As many people are aware, this type of direct, relationship medical practice delivery model concept is still relatively new. The greatest amount of data compiled to date on the loyalty or renewal rates of Concierge Medicine Patients year after year tells us that these practices have an annual renewal rate of about 90.%. Additionally, these types of practices are mainly considered Hybrid business models, which means these doctors and their offices accept insurance and charge an annual retainer fee to their Patients for enhanced access. This number is based on data representing approximately 100,000 Patients nationally.

Retention figures inside concierge medical care practices have proven consistent since the year 2000 but sources have informed us that these retention numbers are slowly declining due to one major factor — some doctors are over-promising and under-delivering. This in turn, leaves the Patient unsatisfied. On the positive side, Patients leaving their concierge care physician are overwhelmingly still choosing Concierge Medicine medical care — albeit just from a different physician in their geographic area.

Long term data on these particular kinds of Patients is currently still being compiled but data supporting the cost effectiveness and affordability of these healthcare models is intriguing. According to various physician journals, a Patient will remain a Patient of a traditional primary care doctor in a typical family practice or general medicine practice, barring an altering event (like a geographic move, death, loss of job, or other unforeseen circumstance) for 5-7 years.

Based upon the data listed above, it appears that retainer medicine or boutique physicians that have a long, relational-history with their Patients are reporting higher retention levels that exceed traditional primary care and family practice expectations. This data, combined with the fact that this model of medicine provides for closer communication and relationship with people, causes us to expect that the majority of Patients will continue to remain with a retainer-based practitioner longer than seven to nine (7-9) years.

The information provided here gives more evidence that these types of medical practices are not just for the deep-pocketed executive. In fact, we have recently learned that over 50% of these types of healthcare consumers make a combined household income of less than $100,000 per year.

All of this data should be very encouraging to the public, as well as the practicing physician anywhere in America. This concept, initially thought of by many as healthcare for the rich — is now accessible and very affordable for couples, seniors on Medicare, young families and individuals.

Direct Care and Concierge Medicine Fees Remain Fixed, Despite Rising Demand

Citing an improving U.S. economy, we estimate that by 2016, the cost of Concierge Medicine and DPC services may only slightly increase to reflect inflation in approximately eleven U.S. states by less than 2 percent.

We also find that memberships and renewals at hundreds of Concierge Medicine and DPC health clinics across the U.S. remain strong at approximately 93 percent (data collected between 2011 – 2013), despite the effects of the Affordable Care Act and brand-biased by some of its critics.

Since the overwhelming majority of Concierge Medicine and direct pay style medical clinics cater to those who cannot afford high health insurance premiums, these types of medical practices across the nation are now being seen as the most accessible, affordable and best options for Patients who are used to paying large health plan premiums. Couple a Concierge Medicine physician or DPC doctor with a catastrophic care [insurance] plan and you have got a marriage made-in-medicine.

Furthermore, the California HealthCare Foundation Health says some health plans may see a market opportunity through the Exchanges by coupling DPC with a high-deductible wraparound policy that promises to deliver a lower price than conventional insurance products. They cite that Cigna and Associated Mutual are early adopters of this strategy.

Patients are encouraged to be insured by a PPO, HSA, Medicare or a major medical plan in the event of a hospitalization or other catastrophic event adds one physician in the Dallas, TX area. He continues to add, this allows for coverage of services provided outside of our offices and for specialist services to be billed to the Patient's insurance company.

We have reported that in most DPC and concierge medical offices, they do not typically accept health insurance, instead opting to serve Patients in exchange for a recurring monthly fee — usually $50 to $130 — for a defined set of clinical services.

Despite Hollywood's vision and the thought that only high-powered executives use Concierge Medicine, people of all ages and household income are using this brand of medicine across the country.

Large networks of doctors who have modeled their medical practice after these business strategies have claimed a significant portion of the market share and thus help to keep prices from inflating too high in major metropolitan markets.

Various media reports and confirmed sources, including our own, estimate that the average cost for a DPC or a Concierge Doctor is between $725-$2,400 per Patient, per year. Additionally, the average Patient or consumer of Concierge Medicine and DPC services may experience a small annual premium increase of about $25 to $160 per year, in keeping with inflation.

The problem with raising prices for Concierge Patients, especially in private, direct care medicine clinics is that it causes Patients to reassess how much value this care brings to their life, their financial commitment, their current quality of life, past experiences with the doctors' staff, traffic and travel interruptions and how often they actually utilize services on an annual basis.

We receive regular inquiries from Doctors who are looking at how much they are charging for services. These Physicians are attempting to determine how they can balance those fees and still charge what their Patients will pay without appearing to price-gouge their Patients. They are also trying to analyze how the Affordable Care Act is affecting and will affect their Patient-base in the future.

"The doctor of the future will no longer treat the human frame with drugs, but rather will cure and prevent disease with nutrition."
-Thomas Edison

Earlier Hours Inside "Modern" Medical Practices Becoming The Norm

If your mornings are anything like most, you prefer to schedule the majority of your health exams and check-ups right away. In fact, the earlier the better! Many will take the first possible appointment or even the second visit of the day because they know that their physician(s) are revving up for a busy day — and they need to get their day moving.

These are big fans of practices which cater to the Patient with hours starting at 6:30am or even 7am. Just last week, I personally visited a concierge practice in North Atlanta area and was pleasantly surprised at the early morning or after 6pm appointments. They have made available to their Patients every Monday, Tuesday and Thursday. Flexible appointment times make your practice more appealing to Patients with busy schedules.

"To be able to practice in this fashion, the patient roster is limited to a maximum of 600 patients," says Dr. Andrea Klemes is the Chief Medical Officer of MDVIP. "Each patient enjoys a 90- to 120-minute annual wellness visit similar to an executive style physical. This includes an exam, review and coaching for every patient. Follow up visits last 30 minutes. Under this calculation, doctors see eight to 12 patients a day. Physicians benefit on multiple fronts. We enjoy financial stability in this uncertain time. We regain the freedom to practice the way we were trained. Our time, tools and technology improve our abilities and make us even more valuable to our patients than we were before. Partnering with a consultant or an organization that provides the resources to transition successfully to this model is critical particularly to ensure that your practice is compliant with all federal and state laws. The model even improves national outcomes. Hospitalizations are down – by 79% in Medicare patients in one year and 72% in commercial patients. Readmission rates for common problems (Acute MI, CHF and pneumonia) are all under 2%, as compared to the national averages that range from 15% to 21%. Control of chronic conditions is better against all benchmarks and together, these saved the healthcare system over $300 million a year. The patient benefits of a smaller size practice include same-day appointments, 24-hour availability, no waiting and a higher level of coordination of care. As a result, patient satisfaction tops 94%, with nine in 10 patients renewing annually. Moreover, physician satisfaction is over 95%. With the right tools and model, we get to practice medicine the way we had been trained. We find the time to talk. We tease out buried details, identify issues, and become the hands-on healers we once were. For their part, patients become more accountable and see real results."

"A business is successful to the extent that it provides a product or service that contributes to happiness in all of its forms."

-Mihaly Csikszentmihalyi

Five Ways To Keep Your Staff Happy As Your Concierge Practice Grows

Most Concierge Doctors and DPC physicians are looking to grow their practices after the second or third year. The first year has it is challenges but it is more about stabilizing the new Patient members, proving the pricing model locally and making several much needed adjustments internally. But about the 18-month mark, we have learned that a Physician's success hits and it hits fast. So, how can you scale your medical practice without shedding the shared values and culture that helped make you successful in the first place?

Here are a few ways that you can keep your Concierge Medical and DPC practices small business values as your local clinic continues to grow:

1. Keep a local doctors/business owner's perspective. When you initially change your business or pricing model to a Concierge Medicine or DPC practice, it is easy to empathize with the pains felt by your Patients. Empathy is important in more than just Patient support. You will also need your employees to all be able to step inside the small medical practice owner's loafers or heels and focus on how to make your Patient's lives easier.

2. Build an internal philosophy of shared, common beliefs. As many industry insiders will tell you, staff and spousal belief in the new business model is more important than signing a new Patient. But why? *Concierge Medicine Today* (CMT) has interviewed physician after physician in many major markets and found that the results are the same. If you have even just one staff member in your practice that does not think Concierge Medicine or your DPC pricing structure is a good idea – that this bad attitude will actually begin to lose you Patients, revenue and your reputation.

The solution, find the bad apple (if you have one that is) and either reposition them to employment in the practice where direct Patient interaction is not required or ask them to potentially move on to another place of employment. Every small medical practice, particularly in Concierge Medicine or DPC has its own culture. It does not mean that all of your employees must think exactly the same way as you do. But by creating a set of shared beliefs, belief in your new business and pricing model, forecasted goals and celebrated achievements internally causes everyone employed to have the same idea for how to accomplish their daily tasks, set priorities, make decisions, treat Patients, and treat each other.

3. Involve your spouse or at the very least, keep them tuned-in on your accomplishments at the practice. Many physicians and their spouses work together in the same office. *The Concierge Medicine Research Collective* (April 2013), found in the practices surveyed and of the doctors interviewed that – changing your business model to one that is concierge or fee-for-care requires the joint agreement of both spouses, whether they work together or not. This is critical for the practice to succeed after month 18. If your spouse is not in agreement with the change, a transition to a concierge medical practice is not typically recommended by many consultants. It may handicap the emotional state of the physician and ultimately the practice after the first year.

4. Create open channels of communication. *Concierge Medicine Today* has reported since 2010 that the majority of Concierge Medicine practices and DPC clinics employ 1-2 people inside the practice (approx. 62%). When your practice is small everyone wears multiple hats and experiences the practice from multiple facets. As a concierge medical practice grows, communication among staff can become a maze and employees get pigeonholed into certain roles. So a unique approach to keep a small practice buzzing is to make sure everyone (doctor included) rotates through various positions within the practice from time-to-time, whether it is the service window or in the exam room, when possible – remaining HIPPA Compliant of course. A Patient might get the RN one day or an administrative accountant the next day. This unique approach we have learned gives the impression to Patients that this is a family business and everyone is friendly and capable. This unorthodox approach also forces everyone within the practice to stay close to the Patients.

5. Develop your Concierge Medicine practice culture outside of normal office hours. If you expect your employees to love your Patients, your practice must show love to your staff. To do this, it is been suggested that doctors or owners of the practice build-in each year staff activities outside of the practice. For example, one day every year, take a scheduled work day off and take the entire practice staff (and their families if possible) on a group trip (a sporting event, volunteer opportunity like Habitat For Humanity or similar, amusement park, etc.) or take them out to dinner. Typically the best times to do this are not around Thanksgiving or Christmas (but those are important too), but suggested to be in March, May and October. Happy employees treat your Patients better.

Keeping a small concierge medical practice or DPC business culture in your practice as it grows will help you keep practice strong and your employees happy.

Why OB/GYN Concierge Medicine Specialty Is Likely To Succeed.

Many American women aren't seeing an internist or family physician for primary care needs but instead are receiving primary care services from a gynecologist. A lot of women feel comfortable with this because for one, they have found that tests many times overlap. OBGYNs can also be very thorough, women like that.

Under the law, women can select OB/GYNs as their primary care provider and cannot be required to seek a referral or prior authorization to see an in-network OB/GYN specialist. Parents can select a pediatrician as their child's PCP.

Dr. Ira Mickelson of a Detroit, MI practice says the majority of his Patients use him as their primary care doctor, "If we are going to be good physicians we need to be aware of that and take care of all of their needs." Dr. Mickelson continues to say the trend is toward using OB/GYNs for primary care. Some medical schools are even preparing new doctors for this expanded role.

He explained, "Instead of just delivering your babies and pap smears and birth control, we are now thinking more in the lines of total Patient care." So that means an EKG and chest x-ray when appropriate. And a full complement of lab tests, "We always take their blood pressure and we have discussions on quality of life which includes making life healthier."

The cholesterol test Dr. Mickelson uses, the VAP, is even more complete than the one some internists call for, "It gives us a breakdown of the different types of LDL, different types of cholesterol." If a woman is considering using her gynecologist for primary care, she needs to have a conversation about her expectations.

Dr. Mickelson recommends asking the doctor, " 'Are you going to be my primary care doctor, are you going to do my cardiovascular, the rest of my health care, or do I need to find someone else?' I think that needs to be said." Dorothy, a Patient of Dr Mickelson is very happy with just seeing a gynecologist for her annual checkup. She thinks other women would be too. "It is almost like going to the grocery store, one stop shopping and they like that and I think that is why more women today do that."

To answer the question, can an OB/GYN last more than three years in a hybrid concierge practice? The answer is a resounding yes. It might be a different story if insurance was NOT involved or accepted in the practice as the majority of Patients seeking out a concierge physician are concerned about:

- Insurance and/or Medicare participation;
- Price;
- Location.

According to Scott MacStravic, PhD, he writes ... 'The initial concierge practices were all in primary care specialties–family practice, internal medicine, pediatrics–but there are a growing number that are in secondary specialties: 45+ by my count, including "addiction medicine," cardiology, dermatology, general surgery, gynecology, and oncology just to name a few. These specialty practices usually offer the same immediate access, longer appointments, and a proactive health focus as primary care concierge practices. Some also offer home visits. Specialists usually limit their practices to a smaller number of Patients–150-300 compared to the more typical 500-600 Patients for primary–and they more often deal with Patients who already have a chronic condition to be treated.'

*"Work for something because it is good,
not just because it stands a chance to succeed."*

-Vaclav Havel

The Anti-Aging Side Of Concierge Medicine Boosts Patient Retention For The Modern Medical Home.

Concierge Medicine and DPC has evolved to more than just 24/7 care. More Internal Medicine and Family Concierge Doctors are taking a medical home approach — offering added-value services and wellness professionals to focus on anti-aging and medical home solutions. The benefit: concierge doctors are seeing two and three times more Patient's foot-traffic in various markets across the country.

We have asked Concierge and DPC physicians across the U.S. about what makes their practice so popular. Our analysis of this information has concluded that three out of every eight Concierge Medicine and DPC doctors are incorporating anti-aging solutions inside their practice. Concierge and DPC doctors are also incorporating a vast number of other added-value services for Patients such as: Heart burn and gastrointestinal disorders; B12 injections; Vitamin deficiencies; Hormone balancing therapies; Mole checks; Testosterone injections; Medically supervised fat loss programs and a diverse collection of other wellness-focused and anti-aging solutions.

As a DPC or Concierge Doctor, the true value of a practice revolves around the service the doctor and staff provide 24/7 and the relationship they have with each Patient. Concierge Medicine and DPC Doctors work tirelessly at this so as to increase the amount Patients who walk through the door each and every week. This increases Patient retention year after year which we have found since 2009 to present an average of between 90% and 94% Patient retention inside a Concierge Doctors office. So why are Patients choosing Concierge Medicine and DPC care year after year across the country in droves? Interviews and surveys from both doctors and Patients by our staff say it is because of: the service they provide; the transparent pricing structure; and the relationship with a 24/7 physician who does not have to look at a chart to know their name. But keeping Concierge Medicine Patients coming back healthier and happier year after year can be a significant challenge if the right relationship and service just isn't there.

"I give a lot of B12 injections and testosterone injections for those who need it," says Dr. Sarah Mildred Gamble, D.O. of Greenwich, CT who runs a thriving Concierge Medicine practice. "I also do a lot of in office procedures like mole checks and removal, trigger point injections ... and then there are my Botox/fillers appointments too."

We are also learning that the Concierge Medicine and DPC clinics that are introducing anti-aging service and a medical home philosophy in their local markets are seeing Patient foot traffic double or even triple in each and every age group from six to sixty.

"I give a lot of B12 injections and testosterone injections for those who need it. "I also do a lot of in office procedures like mole checks and removal, trigger point injections ... and then there are my Botox/fillers appointments too."

Dr. Sarah Mildred Gamble, D.O. of Greenwich, CT who runs a thriving Concierge Medicine practice.

"Many of my female Patients choose for me to perform their annual OB/GYN [gynecology] exam, but those who have their own gynecologist follow up with them," writes Dr. Alexa Faraday to Concierge Medicine Today. "What I found interesting was that when I left my old practice — I had a 10% Medicare population. That fraction has grown to almost half, suggesting to me that some of the folks most interested in this model are older Patients."

Dr. Alexa Faraday is a Board Certified Physician in Internal Medicine operating a successful Concierge Medicine practice based in Baltimore, MD.

The Anti-Aging Side Of Concierge Medicine Boosts Patient Retention For The Modern Medical Home (Con't)

We learned that three out of every eight Concierge Doctors were incorporating unique anti-aging and medical home solutions into their practice across the U.S. in 2012 and 2013. These doctors are by choice and nature, treating nearly 90% of their Patient's healthcare concerns, ailments and needs each year. But that relationship can get repetitious year after year so doctors are adapting. They are hearing what is successful from their own Patients and finding out what is appealing to their audience and local marketplace because the Concierge and DPC doctors are actually communicating with their Patients more often.

The public loves the idea of Concierge Medicine and DPC or loathes it. If they truly understand it, there is nothing that quite compares to it. But it is an educational curve that we are slowly overcoming in the marketplace nationally here at *Concierge Medicine Today*. Since the election of November 2012, we have seen a tremendous increase in the amount of interest, inquiries and physician searches across the U.S. People are concerned about the Affordable Care Act, access to physicians and unsure about costs.

"In some respects, our well-heeled patient population and their inherent and unique needs is our specialty. We are fortunate to have interesting and distinguished patients; I cherish the relationships deeply," said MD² founder Dr. Howard Maron.

The anti-aging and medical home delivery model fits well inside a Concierge Medicine and DPC practice. The nutritional component, the wellness solutions, the anti-aging and team-focused health care delivery professionals led by a Concierge or DPC Doctor are providing comprehensive and continuous health care services to Patients. They simply cannot find all of these services in one place elsewhere. This combination is increasing Patient retention and Patient interest in the concept. The goal here is healthy outcomes for Patients followed by increased Patient retention outcomes for the Physician year after year.

"Many of my female Patients choose for me to perform their annual OB/GYN gynecology exam, but those who have their own gynecologist follow up with them," writes Dr. Alexa Faraday to Concierge Medicine Today. Dr. Faraday is a Board Certified Physician in Internal Medicine operating a successful Concierge Medicine practice based in Baltimore, MD. "What I found interesting was that when I left my old practice — I had a 10% Medicare population. That fraction has grown to almost half, suggesting to me that some of the folks most interested in this model are older Patients."

Dr. Shira Miller runs a Concierge Holistic Medical Practice in southern California that focuses specifically on anti-aging and Menopause. It is very popular. So popular in fact, she's become 'Facebook's Most Popular Menopause Doctor.'

"I work to ensure 100% of Patients... visit at least once per year," said Dr. Miller. "When Mother Nature quits, I'm here to help you keep your [the Patient's] mind, body, and sex life healthy as you age."

"The anti-aging and medical home delivery model fits well inside a Concierge Medicine and DPC practice environment. The nutritional component, the wellness solutions, the anti-aging and team-focused health care delivery professionals led by a Concierge and DPC Doctor are providing comprehensive and continuous health care services to Patients. They simply cannot find all of these services in one place elsewhere. This combination is increasing Patient retention and Patient interest in the concept. The goal here is healthy outcomes for Patients followed by increased Patient retention outcomes for the Physician year after year."

-Catherine Sykes, Author, Speaker,
Healthcare Strategist

Self-Serve Beverage Stations Making Big Impression With Concierge/DPC Consumer

Occasionally a Patient might run out of their house without your hot cup of tea or favorite blend of coffee at their side.

The Keurig and K-Cup coffee makers and other single-serve and pod coffee/tea brewers have come into businesses with a flurry of excitement over the past two years. Patients spending any amount of time in your office will appreciate the convenience and freshness. Employees of Concierge Medical and D{C practices love the easy, no mess, clean-up they provide.

In recent months, these single coffee cup brewers have become much more affordable and stylish. Some of the larger big-box wholesale clubs even sell such devices to their members with 60 or more K-Cups included with the price of the coffee maker. So, if you have the traditional-style coffee maker which involves making a full pot of coffee, you are way behind the trend...!

*"Listen to counsel and accept discipline,
That you may be wise the rest of your days."*

~Proverbs 29:11 NIV

Chapter 7 –
Running With The Giants.
Expert Advice and Lessons Learned From Some of Today's Most Successful Concierge Medicine, DPC Doctors and Industry Leaders.

Running a business is tough. Running a business as a Physician and treating Patients is tougher. But there are some things in business and healthcare you simply cannot learn by reading a book. Here is some of the Concierge Medicine and DPC industry's leading Physician experts and lessons they have learned over the years.

Expert Advice and Lessons Learned From Some of Today's Most Successful Concierge Medicine, DPC Doctors and Industry Leaders.

Dr. Erika Bliss, MD, FAAFP
Qliance (Seattle Location)
509 Olive Way, Suite 1,607
Seattle, WA 98101-1721
Office: 206-913-4700
www.qliance.com

Question: Describe some of the greatest hurdles you and your team have faced over the years and how Qliance overcame those challenges.

Dr. Erika Bliss: "From the beginning, we struggled to communicate to the insurance companies what it is we were trying to do. Initially, during the 2007 Washington State legislative session where we worked with the legislature to coin the term "DPC" and define it as <u>not</u> being insurance, the insurance companies came out strongly against us, claiming that we were going to somehow cherry pick the healthiest people, and drop them when they became sick."

"We spent a lot of time meeting with the insurance commissioner and his staff helping them understand that primary care is for everyone, and that we provide primary care no matter what a person's health profile or situation, and when they are very sick or even terminal (like with cancer or end-stage renal disease), that is one of the most critical times to have a primary care provider who is paying attention to the whole person. In the legislation, we agreed willingly to prohibitions against discriminating against people based on health status (which we never planned to do in the first place). Since we were not trying to be insurance, we had no need to risk stratify, like the insurance companies do. The insurers also took offense to our stance that insurance is not designed to pay for common, predictable, low-cost services such as primary care, and that using it to do so warps the insurance system and sets up the wrong incentives. They took it as us saying that people do not need insurance at all, which is never what we said, we just said you do not need it for primary care. However, from the beginning we told them that our model would help them drive down the cost of claims and would help them keep their premiums competitive. That definitely fell on deaf ears at the time."

"Since the recession and the ACA, though, things have really changed. Now we find ourselves in much more productive discussions with many insurers, and in fact one of them thought DPC had sufficient potential to move them to invest in our company (Cambia/Regence Blue Shield). We have figured out how to submit shadow claims without having to do visit coding at the point of care, so now they can look at what we are doing and compare it to claims from traditional fee-for-service providers and thereby measure the impact we have on downstream claims. However, all of the major carriers are struggling with how to include DPC in their networks, in terms of plan design and IT accommodations."

"There is one plan in the country that I know of that is custom-designed to wrap around DPC, called the Employer Health Ownership Plan, offered by Physician Care Direct and Qliance in collaboration with Roundstone Insurance. This is what is called a "group captive" plan, one that brings together a group of small to medium sized employers (roughly 50-500 employees) to pool risk. The plan offers DPC as the primary care core offering and is structured and priced to recognize the value delivered by the DPC model. We are launching the plan this week, and will be joined by two other independent primary care networks (Family Care Network and Puget Sound Family Physicians), offering geographic coverage from Bellingham to Tacoma."

"The other big opportunity for DPC is to get involved with managed care plans, such as Medicaid managed care and Medicare Advantage. Those carriers often have the infrastructure in place to pay capitated rates, and have some experience with the results you can get when you pay sufficiently for great primary care. We currently work with Coordinated Care, a subsidiary of Centene Corporation in Washington, where we provide Medicaid enrollees with the DPC medical home model. Coordinated Care was also approved to have a plan on the state exchange, so we will start to get some experience with individuals in the commercial market as well."

"I hope that we will see more and more creative plan design that includes innovations like DPC. It will unlock the great potential of this model by making it easier to buy for both individuals and employers, which will in turn inspire more providers to convert their practices."

"I made the switch many years ago into Concierge Medicine, or at least a form of it, and I couldn't be happier. I can provide better care and build a strong relationship with my Patients. It definitely can be challenging since I make myself available 24/7 however, if you can develop a good support structure of other like-minded MDs you can maintain a successful business with less stress than a traditional practice."

~Las Vegas Urgent Care Doctor
https://www.facebook.com/24HourVegasDoctor

Question: What advice do you have for others considering moving into Concierge Medicine or DPC?

Dr. Erika Bliss: I would say the following:

1. Do not be afraid to try something new. If we do not try to do things differently, primary care will continue to languish and we will have a harder and harder time attracting people into the field and ensuring that primary care survives for us, our children, and our grandchildren. You do not have to do it all at once, though – a lot of practices are trying to develop a hybrid model, gradually moving more and more of their Patients to the DPC model. It is challenging to do this if you are caring for large numbers of Patients, but practices are finding ways to do it.
2. Talk to people already doing this. There are now several individual providers and larger companies offering DPC who have learned a lot in the process of developing their practices. Some are starting to offer consulting services.
3. Get to know your local employer community: Many of them are looking for ways to direct purchase healthcare and will be interested in talking with you.
4. Ask yourself if the service model is really for you. Most DPC providers make a commitment to be highly available to their Patients. However, with smaller numbers of Patients, that availability is usually pretty manageable. As our founder, Garrison Bliss, has said, in DPC we work for our Patients, and that means we have to treat them like valued customers. It requires a change in culture and habits not just for the providers, but for their entire staff. It also requires changing your systems and procedures which can be disruptive and costly.
5. Plan on demonstrating value. Accountability is the watchword in healthcare and primary care will be no exception to the requirement that healthcare takes responsibility for the quality and outcomes of our care. If you can, set up your systems from the beginning to capture the kind of performance data people are going to want to see, like Patient experience data, disease management outcomes, hospitalization rates, etc.
6. Join the revolution! In my mind, DPC offers the most promising alternative for those of us who are passionate about primary care and healing relationships with our Patients. Being able to take the time you need to do the right thing for Patients is professionally and personally satisfying in a way that has renewed the passion of many, many providers for what they do. And when we talk with students and residents, or when they visit our practices, they feel our positive energy and love for what we do and can imagine themselves being primary care providers as well, which is good for all of us.

"The Qliance model is structured around the notion of time, and just like any relationship, you need time to be able to fully express yourselves, to tell each other your whole story."

-Erika Bliss, MD, FAAFP
Seattle, WA | Qliance

Dr. Edward Espinosa
Buckhead Concierge Internal Medicine
91 W. Wieuca Road NE
Bldg. A Suite 1000
Atlanta GA 30342
Office :: 404-257-5585
www.bcimonline.com

Question: Describe some of the most successful service programs you have implemented into your practice that Patients enjoy and find very unique when compared to other practices.

Dr. Espinosa: Providing courtesy rounds while Patients are hospitalized are beneficial to the Patients in helping them understand their hospitalization in real time and facilitate continuity of care and improve quality of care before, during, and after hospitalization.

Question: During your startup period until now, what are some of the cost saving measures you are implementing/implemented in your practice to help keep your budget on-track?

Dr. Espinosa: Summer hours from 8:30 to 4:00 instead of 8:30 to 5:00 pm helps us reduce payroll costs, particularly as the summer tends to be our slower season.

Question: Describe the top 3 things that now make your Concierge Medicine practice very different from traditional, insurance-based/managed care medical clinics?

Dr. Espinosa: We provide house calls. We provide hospital visits. We provide an application that delivers lab results, medication lists, allergy lists, medical history, etc. to Patient's smartphones.

Question: When Patients ask you about your practice, what are usually the top 3 questions you hear most?

Dr. Espinosa: Does insurance pay for the concierge fee? Will you provide medical care to my children? And What hospitals are you affiliated with?

Question: What have you found is the best way to grow your Patient panel?

Dr. Espinosa: Word of mouth is the best marketing. Request that Patients go online and provide a review.

Question: We have all heard it said, Patient referrals are the best way to educate and encourage new enrollments, particularly as it relates to Concierge Medicine. What Patient referral strategy have you used and has it worked?

Dr. Espinosa: Working as a hospitalist in a local hospital makes a significant difference with regard to referrals.

Question: When looking back on your Start-Up process and some of the most important decisions you made, what would you have done differently?

Dr. Espinosa: Looking back I would have purchased the building we are in instead of renting.

Question: When you think about the do's and don'ts of starting your Concierge Medicine practice, what are some of the most important things you would definitely do again and some of the decisions you wish you could do-over?

Dr. Espinosa: First, do not spend excessive amounts of money on a robust EMR. Consider paper charts, dictation services or a free EMR. Second, when initiating a concierge practice, consider starting off without a brick and mortar building and either do strictly home visits or rent office space PRN. Third, location of a concierge practice will drive your success. If you place a concierge practice in a geographic area that does not support such a practice economically you will likely fail. Fourth, start blogging early. Consider video blogs as well. Next, be realistic with your Patients early on. Clearly lay out benefits and limitations of a concierge practice. You cannot please everyone. Last, consider variations of a concierge or direct pay model. Hybrids tend to provide Patients more options and while they require more administrative effort are more appealing for Patients.

Question: How do you keep your Concierge Medicine practice running smoothly and what advice would you give to others?

Dr. Espinosa: Keep your staff happy. Staff plays a key role in keeping Patients happy. Make sure front office and nursing staff develops a strong relationship with your Patients.

"My vision is to cultivate a personal Patient - doctor relationship amidst a bustling urban community where impersonal professional relationships are the norm. Our practice strives to deliver quality medical care with an emphasis on evidence based medicine, open communication, easy accessibility, and a focus on customer service. These benefits can lead to an overall improvement in how healthcare is delivered and may ultimately improve outcomes."

-Dr. Edward Espinosa
Buckhead Concierge Internal Medicine
www.bcimonline.com

Dr. Tiffany Sizemore-Ruiz, D.O.
Choice Physicians of South Florida
1409 SE 1st Ave
Fort Lauderdale, FL 33316
Office: 954-523-4141
www.ChoicePhysiciansSFL.com

Dr. Tiffany Sizemore-Ruiz states: "Opening a concierge practice was the most difficult thing I have ever done- but the most rewarding. It is funny. In medical school, we think life will be easier as a resident. As a resident, we just cannot wait to "get out" and finally earn a salary. Then, when we are finally finished with training, we look around and go.. "now what?". For me, it was an easy decision to have my own concierge practice, but a tough achievement to follow through on. Running your own practice is one thing. Running a concierge practice is something else. At times I felt like a sales person, attempting to persuade Patients why my unique practice was right for them. Over time, these conversations become less and less frequent and it became more of me being the doctor and less of the salesperson."

"I will, however, offer a few pieces of advice. One, do not get discouraged. These practices can take a very long time to build. But understand, that once a Patient is a concierge Patient, and see how much time you dedicate to them, you can pretty much bet on the fact that they will be loyal to you (and vice versa) for life. My practice is going well, but I am not quite exactly where I want to be in terms of Patient load. Be Patient, they will come. Two, do not underestimate the power of marketing and publicity. There is nothing better than a good website and, in my eyes, nothing worse than a bad one. Remember, for as much as you google things...your Patients will google you. Have a good on-line reputation and presence. Lastly, do not make promises you cannot keep. If you promise physician access 24/7, provide it. No to little wait times? Follow through. If you cannot keep your promises you have, in turn, lost your credibility."

"Be prepared for one heck of a roller coaster ride, but man is it worth it!"

"*Being a good physician is not just about knowing how to diagnose and treat disease. Honestly...that's what books and studying is for. Being a good doctor entails earning the trust of your patients by being honest and forthcoming. It means knowing how to communicate effectively while still remaining sympathetic. It requires you, first and foremost, to be a human being. It honestly bothers me that young doctors feel like they have to "know everything" to be a great physician. Put down the damn book and go talk to your patient. Be a human being. Be a friend. It's really that simple.*"

-*Tiffany Sizemore-Ruiz, D.O.*
Choice Physicians of South Florida
https://www.facebook.com/ChoicePhysicians

Alexa Faraday, M.D.
Greater Baltimore Medical Center (GBMC)
6701 North Charles Street, Suite #4,106
Baltimore, MD 21204
Office: 855-372-5392
www.DrAlexaFaraday.com

Dr. Alexa Faraday states: "I have been practicing internal medicine since 1993, and I was an employed physician until 2011. At that time I decided to start my own concierge internal medicine practice. I am very glad that I made the decision. My practice is now independent of all insurers, including Medicare. Because we are independent, we are able to focus on the needs of our Patients, without insurance restrictions and regulations. Because my practice is smaller, I am able to devote more time and attention to each Patient. The Patients who came with me love it, and they tell me so often, unsolicited, how glad they are that I made the switch. As one Patient said, "Of course I loved you before, but I like this model so much more!" The Patients who joined after my transition were Patients specifically looking for this model. We also have Patients who did not follow with me initially, citing the extra expense, but returned later because they were not satisfied with care they received elsewhere and wanted to come back."

"I am accountable to my Patients and my conscience, and that suits me. My Medicare population increased from 10% to over 40%, an increase that tells me some of the folks most interested in this model are older Patients. But we have many young Patients, including students signed up by their parents, busy professionals, healthy people who want to stay that way, and people with chronic conditions who want a doctor willing and able to manage all of their issues."

"I would make the observation that the people who chose this model are people who value a relationship with their own personal physician, who need some amount of medical care, and who are willing and able to pay for it out of pocket. I daresay any person who had the choice would chose concierge medical care because it offers enhanced access to one's own physician and better service than what is presently available in a traditional medical practice."

"The Patients who came with me love it, and they tell me so often, unsolicited, how glad they are that I made the switch."

~ Alexa Faraday, M.D.
Baltimore, Maryland
www.DrAlexaFaraday.com

Dr. Alexa Faraday continues: "There is no substitute for a doctor who one knows and trusts, and who acts exclusively on behalf of one's own needs and interests. Fortunately, many people can have this type of care. For people who are enrolled in high deductible insurance plans, they can apply their annual retainer fee toward their deductible. For people who have flexible spending accounts, they can use the money from that account toward the annual retainer fee. My fee is less than the cost of a daily sandwich lunch or a monthly cable contract. I think if more of the public were aware of how affordable this care can be, more people would be clamoring for it. Access 24/7, prompt appointments, same or next day sick visits, unhurried visits, health care coaching, continuity and advocacy. What is there not to recommend this model of care?"

Dr. Thomas Lagrelius M.D., F.A.A.F.P.
Skypark Preferred Family Care
23451 Madison Street, Suite 140
Torrance, CA 90505
Office: 310-378-6200
www.skyparkpfc.com

Dr. Thomas Lagrelius states: "Direct practice is growing rapidly in my community and nationally because Patients now realize that joining is about the only way they can have a highly skilled constantly available primary care doctor they can count on 24/7/365 to manage their care in and out of the hospital and give detailed preventive care. In our practices they are treated literally like family members."

"In insurance based practices they are sometimes treated as incidental to the contractual relationship the doctor has with the insuring authority. When Patient care and access is negatively impacted they find this very disturbing. That is when they start looking for one of us. When they experience the huge difference and the relatively low cost of membership, they tell their friends and family. The snowball effect is now obvious."

"All the direct practices in my community, and there are now seven, are busy. Most are full with waiting lists. From 2005 to 2008 I was the only one here. Then a rapid proliferation was seen which I admit I actively promoted. The momentum is now very strong. Several more such practices are in the wings here. On the other hand, doctors fearful of doing direct practice or doubting they can handle 24/7/365 call are running the other way to employment situations. The dichotomy could not be more stark."

"There are basically two ways of looking at health care, the public health model and the Hippocratic model. In the past few decades our society has been moving towards the public health model and away from the classic Hippocratic model. Direct practice is a reaction to that trend. In the public health model the doctor's primary duty is to look at the best interests of the general population. As long as those interests are in line with the interests and needs of an individual Patient all is well. But if they conflict the individual Patient may suffer. Doctors doing this model tend also to be employed rather than independent. In the Hippocratic model the doctors primary duty is to look at the best interests of the one individual Patient he/she is dealing with at the moment pretty much (though not entirely) to the exclusion of the interests of other parts of society. The focus is reversed in order. If those individual interests are in conflict with those of government or payers it is the doctor's duty to advocate for the Patients best interest and not usually for the society as a whole."

"Remaining independent and non-employed by a larger entity seems best suited to this model, though there can be exceptions. One exception that comes to mind is the Virginia Mason Clinic in Seattle which employs Concierge Doctors who behave pretty much like I do."

"These contrasting models lead to entirely different approaches that change doctor Patient relationships and the level of trust completely. Patients in public health model practices sometimes do not trust the system. The public is beginning to get this distinction and for obvious reasons they want the Hippocratic direct practice approach in their own personal care."

"The public health model works well only when government is running clean air and water programs, immunization campaigns etc. It does not work well for Patients seeking their personal best options behind the closed door of the exam room and at the hospital bedside. The irony of the whole issue is that we now have data, thanks to the fantastic study by MDVIP published in the *Journal of Managed Care*, which proves we save more money by doing the Hippocratic direct practice model well than in a public health model structure. This is no surprise to us, but I'm sure it is a shock to the other side."

"You will never regret being a doctor IF you work only for Patients. But if you do not work only for Patients, you will regret your decision in the end."

-Thomas LaGrelius, MD, FFAFP
Skypark Preferred Family Care
Torrance, CA
www.skyparkpfc.com

Jeffrey S. Gorodetsky, M.D.

Stuart, Florida Family Physician
433 East Ocean Boulevard
Stuart, FL 34994
Office: 772-223-4504
www.jeffreygorodetskymd.com

Dr. Jeffrey Gorodetsky states: "In 1990, I opened my Private Family Practice in Stuart, Florida. In December, 2011, after several years of research, I announced my conversion to a Concierge Medical Practice. In an attempt to alleviate any abandonment feelings from my established, large Patient population, I opted for a "hybrid model"."

"My staff and I tried to schedule selected hours for the concierge and non-concierge practice, but found over the first year this was difficult to manage. It also became a challenge to convert my non-concierge Patients to the concierge model, as they were able to continue their relationship with me. Therefore, I made the decision, in January 2013, to restrict my schedule to concierge Patients and those individuals coming to the practice for an initial visit. Two Physician Assistants are assigned the balance of Patients within the practice."

"The conversion process is not an easy one. My staff and I are cognizant of the fact that we must consistently communicate the benefits of this choice in care, with the challenge to increase my concierge numbers and convert my non-concierge Patients. Another issue that I faced was attempting this redesign of the practice following the economic meltdown. Many Patients indicated their hesitancy to an additional expense due to financial considerations."

"With the growth in popularity of the DPC Model, I am now offering new concierge Patients the option of paying their fee either monthly or quarterly, to alleviate the annual lump sum financial burden. I did experience some initial attrition within the first 12 months, however, this second year I am now seeing a growth to my concierge practice."

"From my experience, I recommend that physicians contemplating a hybrid concierge practice restrict their personal Patients to those who have chosen the concierge services, while assigning non-concierge Patients to either another physician, physician assistant or nurse practitioner. Also, the physician and staff embarking on the transition of a current traditional practice or the inception of a new concierge practice must now realize the importance of the role of marketing and sales to their success."

"The conversion process is not an easy one."

-*Jeffrey S. Gorodetsky, M.D.*
Stuart, FL
www.jeffreygorodetskymd.com

Expert Advice and Lessons Learned From Some of Today's Most Successful Concierge Medicine, DPC Doctors and Industry Leaders.

Charles Whitney, M.D.
Revolutionary Health Services
1121 General Washington Memorial Blvd.
Washington Crossing, PA 18977
Office: 215-321-1371
www.RevolutionaryHealthServices.com

Dr. Charles Whitney states: "Shortly after transitioning from my life as a physician in the Air Force into a civilian practice with the University of Pennsylvania, I realized that practicing high-volume medicine was not only burning me out physically, it was taking an emotional toll because I was not able to provide the level of care for my Patients that I wanted to. By 2002 I was contacting friends from residency who were chairs of residency programs, inquiring about joining them in academic medicine. It was during this time that the forward thinkers at University of Pennsylvania presented me with the opportunity to establish their first "boutique" medical practice. I jumped at the chance!"

"Here was a golden opportunity to practice medicine in a way I thought it would be when I finished medical school- After all, didn't most of us go to medical school because we wanted to invest in the lives of our Patients and help to heal the people in our communities? A year later, a business plan change within the PENN organization caused them to abort this pilot program. After a year of experiencing the DPC practice environment there was no turning back for me! I had realized how much I was burning out as the frog in the boiling pot trying to offer my Patients optimal care in time constraints dictated by managed-care. I assumed ownership of the practice and on July 1, 2004 Revolutionary Health Services was born. It has been full speed ahead ever since."

"I personally do not like the term "concierge", as I believe it is perceived as convenience healthcare for the rich and famous. That is not the value we offer. I believe that the movement towards affordable DPC being the predominant financing model in primary care is a movement that MUST happen."

"Financial incentives in the current payment model are backwards. In the traditional financing model, a physician is rewarded for seeing Patients more often in less time, making it more difficult to be accessible and coach them towards health. In the DPC model, a physician is financially rewarded by finding ways to help our Patients create health. We actually see them less the healthier they are. This is why I am currently putting the finishing touches on adding an affordable DPC pricing structure so I can provide optimal care to as many people in my community as possible. I'm even seeking a Medicaid health plan partner to pilot a DPC project in Medicaid Patients. A pilot is being very successfully implemented in Seattle Washington. Proving that DPC can be a successful business model in the Medicaid population will significantly impact our ability to make DPC the predominant financing structure nationwide!"

21st century medicine has many tools available to effectively practice "Third Era Medicine". The third era of medicine is a paradigm shift mindset change where our primary goal as a physician is to empower an intrinsically motivated Patient to create personal health. As physicians, most of us are trapped in a second era mindset of waiting for disease to occur and "manage" it. We have lost the vision to prevent or cure disease. We are happy to wait until a 70% obstruction shows up on a stress test to address heart disease. We do not treat dementia until symptoms begin, at which time it is often too late. Why not *cure* diabetes or hyper tension instead of just manage it? It is only through the personalized medicine platform of DPC that I am able to effectively practice third era medicine- It cannot be practiced in the 6-8 min. office visit of a traditional insurance based medical office!"

"I have taken what I consider to be the best of DPC and third era medicine to create a very innovative business model that I call Third Era Direct™. The cornerstone of my third era direct practice is the utilization of many clinically proven, but underutilized diagnostic tests that give a very clear picture to forecast a person's health trajectory. Data suggesting early disease are very motivating and engage a Patient to take responsibility for their own health. When shown their poor forecast, it forces them to take a realistic look in the mirror at their current health status, and many actually act! They are given a highly individualized action plan based on their personal results."

"No longer do I have to "convince" them to do anything. If time is taken to educate a Patient about the significance of our findings, they usually beg me to coach them about their role to alter their health path. I have taken more Patients off of medication in the past 3 years since implementing this career altering approach than I did in the prior 20 years combined! I'm certain that many heart attacks, strokes, cancers, and even cases of dementia are being prevented. An engaged, motivated Patient will act if taught how to by a caring health care team."

"I love my job! Unfortunately, very few family physicians and internists can say that. To save our profession from extinction given the exodus of medical students to subspecialties, we must offer a physician in a primary care specialty the ability to love their job. What do I love about my job? I love the relationships I nurture with my Patients, I love to problem solve, and I love to coach my Patients to health. All of these take time- Time that is only available in a DPC setting."

"I love my job! Unfortunately, very few family physicians and internists can say that. To save our profession from extinction given the exodus of medical students to subspecialties, we must offer a physician in a primary care specialty the ability to love their job."

- Charles Whitney, M.D.
Washington Crossing, PA | Revolutionary Health Services
www.RevolutionaryHealthServices.com

Expert Advice and Lessons Learned From Some of Today's Most Successful Concierge Medicine, DPC Doctors and Industry Leaders.

Shira Miller, MD
The Integrative Center for Health & Wellness
13749 Riverside Drive, Suite 200
Sherman Oaks, CA 91423
Office: 818-574-8864
www.shiramillermd.com
www.facebook.com/menopausedoctor

Dr. Shira Miller writes: "Most people are not yet used to the idea of paying out-of-pocket for better medicine. Just like all my Patients, I regularly pay out-of-pocket for services which improve my health and the health of my family. So, I try to make sure I do not spend any more than I have to for health insurance. Below I share with you exactly how I now save a lot of money on health insurance every month. And, how you could easily do the same for yourself, your family, and maybe even your employees."

"First off, for many years I have had a low premium/high deductible health insurance plan that is eligible for a Health Savings Account (HSA). Having an HSA is similar to having an extra IRA just for health care and allows me to pay for health care expenses using pre-tax dollars or to save that pre-tax money for future healthcare expenses. But, over the past several years, even the cost of that low premium plan has doubled! Yikes!"

"So, a couple of months ago, I was motivated to search online and make some phone calls to try and get a better deal. The result? I started saving over $200 per month on health insurance. That is a savings of over $2400 per year! And, my annual deductible is $500 less than my previous plan. I do not know about you, but that is not exactly pocket change in my life. I found that for me in California, I got the best deal by switching to an HSA-eligible high deductible/low premium plan through HealthNet. (Yes, I had to join the California Farm Bureau to get their group discount... a little weird but worth it.)"

"Many people I know are paying thousands of dollars per year just in premiums for their health insurance and aren't even going to their doctor or going to their doctor but not getting healthier. Why not reduce the amount you pay in premiums and spend your money on health services that will actually help you get healthy? Or, save the difference for potential future healthcare expenses? Especially for people who are generally healthy and just trying to stay that way, I think getting this type of health insurance really makes sense, even if they have to pay out-of-pocket for much of their medical services. But, please know, I am not recommending you change your current health insurance policy. I am not your financial planner, accountant, or insurance agent. Only you know what health insurance policy is best for you. All I am saying is,

320

research your health insurance options seriously. If you think you are paying more for health insurance than you are actually getting out of it, you may benefit from shopping around for a low premium/high deductible plan."

Dr. Shira Miller continues: "Most people get health insurance for peace of mind about potential future healthcare expenses. But, just having health insurance does not actually improve your health or reduce your risk of chronic diseases. After the age of 60, it is considered "normal aging" to have chronic diseases, whereas "successful aging" is defined as having no chronic diseases and being in good physical and mental health. In fact, a recent study showed that engaging in multiple healthy behaviors makes a person 3 times as likely to age successfully (*CMAJ*, October 22, 2012). So, if you want to have true assurance about your health, invest in getting healthy now. *Being in optimal health is your best policy for reducing the risk of future healthcare expenses from chronic diseases.*"

"In my practice, I focus on health and wellness, not just chronic disease (although I treat those too). This year alone, I have helped my Patients reverse diabetes, reverse overweight or obese, reduce or discontinue antidepressant medications, discontinue heart medications, discontinue thyroid medications, discontinue anti-inflammatory medications, increase their own natural testosterone levels, avoid surgery, reverse the side-effects of menopause, improve their appearance and self-esteem, and more! Is your health insurance policy doing that for you? If not, that is okay. Similar to how auto insurance works, you need to have health insurance in case something really bad happens to you and it is your responsibility to keep yourself healthy. But, you may want to consider paying less for health insurance and paying more for medical services which are actually going to help you achieve optimal health."

"My focus is on being a trusted advisor and I do not want to have any potential conflict of interests. For example, a lot of doctors make money on supplements, for me I take that out of the equation. In terms of my practice, I just want to focus on providing the best advice I can give my Patients, not worrying about making money off retail."

-Shira Miller, MD
Sherman Oaks, CA | LA's Menopause and Anti-Aging Doctor
www.shiramillermd.com
www.facebook.com/menopausedoctor

"In terms of Patient discounts, I try to negotiate discounted cash pricing
for my Patients whenever possible. Whether it is for blood testing, radiology,
or supplements/medications - I would rather they keep their money for my know-how/concierge
fees. And a lot of times cash-pricing makes their life easier,
because they do not have to wonder or worry about whether or
not insurance will cover, etc."

-Shira Miller, MD
Sherman Oaks, CA | LA's Menopause and Anti-Aging Doctor
www.shiramillermd.com
www.facebook.com/menopausedoctor

Dr. Robert Nelson
316 W. Main Street
Cumming, GA 30040
Phone: 470-297-8089
robertnelsonmd@encompasshd.com
www.encompasshd.com

Question: Why did you choose to start a DPC practice?

Dr. Robert Nelson: "After working for many years in a healthcare system dominated by bureaucratic insurance networks and burdensome billing regulations, things seemed to be getting steadily more complicated for doctors and Patients. Virtually no one thought it was getting any easier to navigate the increasingly complex, confusing and frustrating system of third-party networks; including Medicare. I had become a de facto employee and glorified bill collector for the third-party payers, as opposed to working directly and solely for the Patient's best interest. I became convinced that I needed to help shape a fundamental reset in the way we deliver and pay for routine medical care."

Question: What do you believe are the greatest benefits to your Patients?

Dr. Robert Nelson: "Simple and direct is better! Working directly for the Patient, as opposed to being a "contracted network provider" is an extremely liberating & satisfying experience, for doctor and Patient alike. Indeed, that one-to-one interaction is the essence of a health working doctor-Patient relationship. I believe that is the way medical care is supposed to be. This kind of unfettered direct engagement between doctor and Patient can never be achieved in a system of third-party networks where the doctor is a "provider" of services paid by someone else and the Patient is relegated to a passive "network subscriber"."

Question: What makes your practice unique?

Dr. Robert Nelson: "My practice is unique in that it takes an old school method of delivery (house calls) and gives it a modern twist. The core driver of the practice is my "Virtual Office". Combined with email communications, the virtual office allows for superior 24/7 communication, rapid triage of medical problems, access to medical records and online payment options for my Patients. My Patients never have to go through a receptionist to get ahold of me; communications are very simple and direct."

Dr. Robert Nelson continues: The other unique feature is that the practice is 100% dedicated to price transparency and all prices are clearly posted on the website. This transparency, combined with a DPC business model, gives very important financial leverage to the Patient-consumer heretofore not available in third-party financed practices. The cost savings of DPC primary care, compared to insurance based primary care, is substantial. Providing mobile-based care, combined with lifestyle-friendly electronic communication methods for my Patients, is a hard combination to beat when it comes to providing good Patient/customer service."

"I believe that is the way medical care is supposed to be. This kind of unfettered direct engagement between doctor and Patient can never be achieved in a system of third-party networks where the doctor is a "provider" of services paid by someone else and the Patient is relegated to a passive 'network subscriber'."

-Dr. Robert Nelson
316 W. Main Street
Cumming, GA 30040
Phone: 470-297-8089
robertnelsonmd@encompasshd.com
www.encompasshd.com

Carrie Bordinko, MD
Consolaré Primary Care
Internal Medicine, CEO
4306 E. Desert Crest Drive
Paradise Valley, AZ 85253
Office: 602-350-2633
www.ConsolareMD.com

Question: What recommendations do you have for residents considering a career in Concierge Medicine?

Dr. Carrie Bordinko: "Gain some customer service experience– try a service industry job as these skills are not taught in med school. Moving into Concierge Medicine is not solely about providing excellent medical care without the restraints of insurance industry mandates. You have to also appreciate the lost art of customer service so long ago forgotten when visiting a healthcare institution. Many times my clients (notice I do not use the word "Patients") have noted why they refer their friends to my practice. It is the attention to detail, always delivering exactly what is promised and then some, and keeping their unique needs positioned first with a flexibility to offer new programs or meet needs as quickly as they are identified. This is the cornerstone of customer service."

"In our practice, if the request falls within the parameters of medical and we do not currently have a solution for a client we simply state, " we do not have a solution for you today but will work on one immediately" and then set a firm time on when the solution will be offered."

"Consumers are reluctant to pay for medical costs as this is the responsibility of their insurance carrier but happy to pay for service."

Dr. Caroline Abruzese
Personalized Healthcare, LLC
800 Mt. Vernon Hwy, NE Suite 160
Atlanta, GA 30328
Office: 404-303-8889
www.mypersonalizedhealthcare.com

On Patient Conversion:

Step 1. Get your head straight.

Dr. Caroline Abruzese: Why are you doing this? Primary care physicians have a right to make a living. Making a reasonable living is not selfish, manipulative, or in conflict with your moral or ethical oaths and obligations as a physician. The practice of medicine is capitalist overhead with socialist reimbursement. I do not know of any other business that has been required to operate under these circumstances. You need to understand the reasons why this is good for you and why this is good for your Patients.

Step 2. Practice answering questions and explaining your model to others.

Dr. Caroline Abruzese: When converting to an annual fee model, Many of us do not like the thought of "selling" or using our position and influence to sway a Patient however, the most important step is expressing to your Patients why you believe this would be a good choice for them. This needs to be done in a tasteful and honest manner and for many of us it takes time and practice to feel comfortable having this conversation. I was such a soft sell that I reassured Patients that it would be fine to change to my partner and bragged about the other doctors willing to take over the remainder of the practice. In an effort to be fair and unbiased, I appeared to lack confidence and undermined my own success.

Step 3. Educate your Patients and know how to say things in many different ways.

Dr. Caroline Abruzese: Consider what elements are most important to express when speaking about an annual fee model and then write out what you want to share in a 2 minute conversation. Patients have different levels of knowledge about finance, what is affordable and feelings about money so explain what the fee is annually and monthly. For example, the annual fee is $1500. and this is equivalent to $125. per month.*

Step 4. Always Ask What They Think.

   Dr. Caroline Abruzese: Leave your ego at the door because people do not like change and will react in many ways. This may be your only opportunity to correct false assumptions so it is important they are invited to be honest and your reaction is important. Remember, this decision is about them even if it feels about you.

   Deciding on whether you will accept the fee to be paid monthly is a big decision. Collecting money can take up a lot of your staff's time. With a few exceptions, I cannot afford to accept monthly payments. If you need to make an exception, I recommend a small processing fee and requiring the payment be made by direct deposit.

Joel Bessmer, MD, FACP
Members.MD
P.O. Box 24822
Omaha, NE 68124
www.members.md
Office: 402-934-6283

Question: Why would someone pursue Concierge Medicine as a career-path?

Joel Bessmer, MD: Concierge Medicine is the way of the future if we want to have a successful primary care system. When you dreamed of becoming a physician, you dreamed of having time to develop a relationship with every Patient to really take care of them—outside of the once-a-year visit, and beyond the notations in their chart.

For a physician who seeks improved Patient outcomes, a concierge practice allows the time to more fully explore underlying causes of illness and disease and have at-length discussions about treatment options or follow-up plans. Because you have the chance to establish a personal relationship with your Patients, they trust you as their personal health adviser. In this way, you can really help them overcome personal barriers to any treatment plan or lifestyle change that is prescribed.

In a concierge practice, you have full control over the length and frequency of your Patients' appointments. This not only allows you to develop a strong relationship with each Patient, but also to truly focus on prevention in your practice. Imagine a 300-lb man with sleep apnea, multiple heart and liver problems who comes in after a knee replacement. He tells you he feels horrible and does not really want to live any more. I spent three hours with him at his first visit. In two weeks, he's lost 16 lbs. and is starting to see the light at the end of the tunnel. Then there is the classic communication—the wife of a Patient who texts me late at night that her husband just cut the tip of his finger and probably needs stitches, can I help? These are the people that Concierge Medicine helps most.

Patients have skin in the game. There is leverage there because they are paying me to tell them what I think and coach them, so they might as well listen.

Question: How did you first get into Concierge Medicine?

Joel Bessmer, MD: I was working at a large academic medical center with many physicians who each took shifts covering the entire Patient population. I realized quickly that when I was not the physician on call, my Patients had to discuss their issues with whoever was available that evening or weekend. I was constantly coming back to find changed treatment plans and confused Patients. This disjointedness broke the intimacy and personal relationship that you develop with your Patients over time. I eventually just stopped using the call service altogether and gave my Patients my personal phone number so they could call me instead of someone they'd never seen before. That was when I realized I needed to practice medicine in a different type of setting so I could truly give my Patients the best possible care.

Question: What was the hardest thing about getting started? How do you feel about that experience now?

Joel Bessmer, MD: I am a pleaser, and starting my own concierge practice was not seen as a positive decision amongst my peers at the academic medical center I left. Personally, there is also a mental aspect of feeling as though you are abandoning a group of Patients. This was difficult at first. However, being an associate program director for a successful internal medicine residency program for 11 years, my passion is to save primary care for the future generation of physicians. The concierge model is a primary care practice that mentors can make attractive to the future generation. To those who say Concierge Doctors are hurting the system by diminishing the number of Patients we can care for, my reply is: if you keep doing the same thing year after year, you are going to get the same results! If we do not focus on salvaging the doctor-Patient relationship and allowing the appropriate time for each Patient's care and follow-up, Patients will begin to feel their primary care is a waste of time. Not to mention that physicians will burn-out faster and faster because a practice that is overcrowded and forcing a physician down to eight-minute appointment times is not sustainable.

Question: What would you do again, or not do, in terms of starting your own concierge practice?

Joel Bessmer, MD: Nothing I can think of, but did we make mistakes? Absolutely. No new business or concept is going to be perfect at roll out. I have learned so much along the way that has helped me to develop the perfect practice.

Question: What other thoughts/tips/challenges can you share with someone thinking about getting started?

Joel Bessmer, MD: Please do not go it alone....seek advice/guidance with those of us that have experience. Make sure you understand the medical legal aspects of this that might be very specific for your state.

Question: How is your practice doing now?

Dr. Joel Bessmer, MD: It is now full. Slow and steady growth is ideal in this type of practice because it allows you to offer Patients a personalized experience. I have found that the "word-of-mouth" aspect (vs. a billboard advertising approach) has been the most consistent factor in building my practice. I consistently have Patients recommending their family members and friends. Getting word of mouth referrals based on high quality care, staff service and Patient satisfaction has been a much more effective tool than traditional marketing. And the slow and steady approach ensures that staff can keep up with new Patients, as opposed to getting a rush of new caseloads that would be more difficult to manage all at once.

"Direct [medical] practices should be successful in most cities and states where there is an inadequate supply of primary care physicians. Most important, a physician needs to have social skills to sell him/herself and the new practice model to their Patients and their community."

-Chris Ewin, MD, FAAFP
One To One, MD, P.A.
5801 Oakbend Trail, Suite 260
Fort Worth, Texas 76132
Office: 817.423.5121
www.121md.net

James Pinckney II, M.D.
Diamond Physicians
8222 Douglas Avenue, Suite 700
Dallas, TX 75225
Office: 214-395-3491
www.diamondphysicians.com
www.Facebook.com/diamondprivatephysicians

Question: How do you define personalized medicine?

Dr. James Pinckney II: Personalized medicine utilizes cutting edge technology such as molecular analysis, ultra-sensitive sonogram, and genotyping to achieve optimum medical outcomes in the management of a Patient's disease or disease predisposition.

Personalized medicine is also known as direct medicine which provides direct access to a private physician 24/7. Direct medicine bypasses inefficient "middle men" to deliver personalized, high-quality medical care. Diamond Physicians is a group of family medicine doctors in Dallas, TX who personalize medical treatment plans for their clients via a state of the art physical exam known as the Diamond 360. The Diamond 360 Advanced Physical Exam embodies personalized medicine by utilizing genetic testing, inflammatory testing, and ultra-sensitive carotid sonogram to determine ones risk for heart attack and stroke. Medical data compiled from the Diamond 360 exam allows Diamond Physicians to tailor a customized medical treatment plan for their clients.

Question: What does the current landscape of personalized medicine look like?

Dr. James Pinckney II: Personalized medicine is gaining momentum in response to sprawling waste and frustration with healthcare delivery systems. Second, Personalized medicine will provide greater knowledge of Patient's genetic risk. Lifestyle and nutrition will play a monumental role in reducing risk of disease. Treatment decisions will improve secondary to higher levels of Patient education.

Question: Is it catching on or are stakeholders finding it too expensive to deliver the necessary technologies to determine the best treatment/medications for individuals?

Dr. James Pinckney II: Preventative medicine is now our top priority. The upfront costs associated with genetic testing, inflammatory testing, etc. pales in comparison to the cost of treating chronic disease. Stakeholders are realizing that it is more important to invest in technologies that detect disease at an earlier stage when it is less challenging to treat effectively. Spending capital now on tailored treatment plans for individuals will save billions in the future.

Question: How are these therapies developed?

Dr. James Pinckney II: As a direct medicine physician who implements customized medical treatment for each client, my knowledge in regards to the development of actual therapies is limited. We perform genetic tests to tailor therapy, but do not develop the actual test.

Question: What are the benefits/challenges of personalized medicine? How well are they working thus far?

Dr. James Pinckney II: Personalized Medicine detects disease much earlier than traditional medicine. It enables Diamond Physicians to select optimal therapy reducing trial-and error prescribing and reducing adverse drug reactions. We believe it increases Patient compliance with therapies while shifting the emphasis in medicine from a reactive approach to a proactive or preventative approach. Last, it reduces the overall cost of healthcare.

There are challenges however. Convincing the general public to frequent their physician at least once a quarter even when they are not sick. We need to change the perception of society from reactive to proactive. We must make lifestyle modifications before you are diagnosed with hypertension, hyperlipidemia, or diabetes to achieve the best medical outcome.

Question: What do insurers think about personalized medicine? Will they cover the diagnostic technologies as well as the medications themselves?

Dr. James Pinckney II: Right now it is challenging to attain insurance coverage for diagnostic technologies performed on completely healthy individuals. The current system requires disease to be present for coverage to be obtained which is unfortunate. Patients should be rewarded for pursuing personalized medicine and obtaining reassurance that they are in good health, not penalized. Insurers should be ecstatic about personalized medicine, since millions in insurance claims will be eliminated secondary to prevention of chronic disease.

Question: What is the reaction of physicians to personalized medicine? Of Patients? Are the latter willing to pay for it?

Dr. James Pinckney II: Physicians are enthusiastic at the potential to treat disease at an earlier stage. Diamond Physicians are family medicine doctors and our goal is to improve the quality of life of our Patients by preventing chronic disease. Our clients love our model, and are thrilled at the opportunity to seize control of their health. They are 100% willing to pay for exemplary healthcare and access to the latest disease detecting technologies.

Question: For what diseases are there likely to be targeted therapies?

Dr. James Pinckney II: There are emerging target therapies for hypertension, atherosclerosis, coagulation disorders, Non-Hodgkin's lymphoma, AML leukemia, breast and lung cancer

"In selecting only a small population of clients and providing dedicated counseling sessions, sometimes as often as weekly, allows clients to actively participate in their care plan and to move goals forward at a real-time pace. This enables all of us to realize that healthcare can be a positive experience."

-Dr. Carrie Bordinko
Paradise Valley, AZ | Consolaré Primary Care
www.ConsolareMD.com

Dr. Clint Flanagan and Dr. David Tusek
Nextera Healthcare
8308 Colorado Blvd, Suite 200
Firestone, CO 80504
Office: 303-501-2600
www.nexterahealthcare.com
https://www.facebook.com/NexteraHealthcare/

Designing Our Practice, Nextera Healthcare in Firestone, CO

According to North Vista Medical Center and Nextera Healthcare Co-Founders Drs. Clint Flanagan and David Tusek, "The DPC model was very attractive to us because, under this approach, we could sustain the value of the Patient/provider relationship and create more accessible care for our Patients. We wanted to restore the 'art' of healthcare delivery and not focus just on the science of it. We are credited with being one of the first to market in Colorado with a DPC program via Nextera Healthcare.

An in-depth analysis of our financials revealed we needed to continue operating under the fee-for-service model for their insured Patients, and then introduce the DPC option alongside. We did not want to undermine our existing Patient relationships by declining traditional insurance, but we also wanted a tangible option for Patients who were uninsured or under-insured and forced to seek alternatives due to rising healthcare costs."

Determining the right price point for the monthly DPC membership, and what services would be included in said membership were both of vital importance. At first we considered charging a monthly fee accompanied by a very low fee per office visit. However, we both agreed the dual fee structure would create complexities and we were trying to simplify the delivery of primary care. Thus, we set a $99 per month individual price, $139 per month for couples, $179 per month for a four-person family, and $39 per month per child for additional dependents.

Designing Our Practice, Nextera Healthcare in Firestone, CO (Con't)

We were fortunate to be uniquely qualified to handle a broad range of healthcare issues due to our extensive training in both family and emergency medicine. Thus, the services covered by our monthly membership fee were equally wide-ranging:

- Routine pediatric care
- Adult medicine and wellness
- Gynecological care, including Pap tests
- Care and treatment for chronic conditions, such as high blood pressure and diabetes
- Dermatological services, including treatment and/or removal of precancerous and certain cancerous lesions, cryotherapy and removal of warts, skin tags, age spots and cysts, and acne treatment
- Acute care for non-life threatening emergencies and medical problems
- Wound repair, including stitches or surgical glue
- Fracture care, including casts and splints for broken bones not requiring surgery
- Trigger-point and cortisone joint injections
- Annual physicals
- End-of-life care
- Customized weight management
- Treatment of depression, anxiety and mood disorders
- ADD and ADHD evaluation and management
- Smoking cessation and alcohol abuse management

Our fee also included some critical relationship-building elements that would set us apart, such as (1) unrestricted visits with providers at our three North Vista Medical Center locations; (2) extended office hours, including Saturdays; and (3) remote or virtual access to providers via email or phone.

Due to the additional benefits provided to our Nextera Healthcare members, we created a staff education program on how to handle traditional fee-for-service Patients and DPC members concurrently based on their health issues. Because DPC members were promised round-the-clock access, more urgent Patient issues meant DPC members took priority over fee-for-service Patients. Also, if DPC members needed urgent care after regular office hours, the on-call provider would meet them at a North Vista Medical Center facility for care. Fee-for-service Patients might visit a 24-hour urgent care facility, in contrast. Staff understanding of the flow of their system was critical to fulfilling our promise to our Nextera Healthcare Patients.

Designing Our Practice, Nextera Healthcare in Firestone, CO (Con't)

We also had to acknowledge that, while our services were extensive, certain activities couldn't be performed at North Vista Medical Center. We have always believed in being a Patient's 'healthcare quarterback,' so we negotiated highly competitive rates for lab and imaging services within our market. We determined the services most crucial to our Patients, educated ourselves about available resources in our community, and created a list of options with full cost transparency. A sampling of rates follows:

- CBC $5
- CMP $5
- HgbA1C $11
- Lipid panel $5
- Uric acid $5
- Vitamin D$28
- Ferritin $8
- TSH $8
- Cardio CRP $16

The cost savings we achieved for our Patients was tremendous, thanks to our long-standing community and business relationships. For example, the combined costs of the above tests would be $630 for a self-pay Patient, yet our rates meant all tests combined would cost a Nextera Healthcare member just $91 out-of-pocket.

We negotiated similar discounts for imaging services, as follows:

- MRI non-contrast $450
- MRI with contrast $650
- Athrogram $650
- CT without contrast $300
- CT with contrast $400
- CT with both $450
- Ultrasound $190
- Ultrasound - vascular $250
- Ultrasound - pelvic $250
- Ultrasound – breast $100
- Upper GI $130
- Barium swallow $90
- X-ray - 2 to 3 views $60
- X-ray – 4-plus views $90

Designing Our Practice, Nextera Healthcare in Firestone, CO (Con't)

Ongoing analysis also helped us understand what staffing we would require to accommodate our DPC membership. We used the following rationale to determine provider staffing levels:

The average family medicine physician has a panel of approximately 3,000 Patients under the fee-for-service model. However, a DPC provider can generate similar revenue with a Patient base of approximately 1,000 members, which reduces Patient volume and increases the amount of time spent with each Patient, a cornerstone of the DPC value proposition. Our DPC model allows us to split shifts. Ideally, four providers work out of one location, with two providers working on weekday mornings, two on weekday afternoons, and two on Saturdays. Under our model, DPC providers work a 30-hour week, far less than the typical fee-for-service primary care provider who works a 50 to 60-hour week.

"Initially, we marketed Nextera Healthcare to uninsured and under-insured individuals as a way to test membership price points, evaluate Patient volume, and collect data on Patient satisfaction. We are now laser-focused on marketing too small to mid-sized businesses that are seeking an affordable employee health benefit that meets the Affordable Care Act (ACA) and enables them to maintain a competitive edge by attracting and retaining top talent. It is that skilled workforce that expects a comprehensive health benefit, and we provide a cost-effective solution. When Nextera Healthcare is paired with a high-deductible health plan for major or catastrophic medical events that might occur outside of primary care – something we recommend – the employer mandate in the ACA is satisfied."

- Dr. Clint Flanagan and Dr. David Tusek
Firestone, CO | Nextera Healthcare

Eugene T. Conte, D.O., FAOCD
Cosmetic Dermatology Associates of Prescott, AZ
212 S. Montezuma Street, Suite 6
Prescott, AZ 86303
Office: 928-515-2359
www.cosmeticdermatologyprescott.com
www.facebook.com/cosmeticdermatologyprescott

Dr. Eugene T. Conte writes: "I have practiced my specialty of Dermatology the "traditional way " for 30 years. It is now time to take the control back that we lost many years ago by not paying attention to what was happening around us. The first thing I did when I came to Prescott Arizona where no one is practicing concierge dermatology. That is right. Practicing, NOT offering, concierge service, is to educate , educate , and educate the public more than to educate physicians. Many Physicians are so set in their ways they will never change."

"No one knows anything except that our current health care system in the United States gives some Patients choices when it comes to care but often these choices are limited to a simple no frills visit, and a quick examination without time for the Patients concerns or questions to be answered. Therefore, Patients have become displeased and frustrated with limited or restricted access to their physician, lower quality of care in some cases, and a lack of customer services from their current health insurance carrier and/ or medical professional, no matter what their medical specialty may be."

"I tell my Patients that ask 'Why does this model work?' My concierge model of service works because it reduces office administrative costs and eliminates the hassle of dealing with insurance billing for both the physician and the Patient. This means the cost of services is reduced and the savings are passed on to the Patient. This benefits all the Patients , whether they use my concierge program or my reduced fee for service program (see my website for details CosmeticDermatologyPrescott.com)."

"I tell Patients this is a perfect model for Patients who choose not to carry health insurance, have a high deductibles on their insurance plans such as MSA's, HSA's or Flex spending accounts or just want more face to face time with their health care provider."

"I tell my Patients that this model becomes a "win-win" for all who are involved. Shortly after I opened my concierge practice in Prescott one of my new Patients said ... 'I really like coming to your office because I do not feel like I am at Disneyland.' I was perplexed by his statement and asked him, 'What do you mean?' He replied, 'It is not a three hour wait and a 20 second ride like it is when I take the kids to Disneyland.'"

-Eugene T. Conte, D.O. FAOCD
Prescott, AZ | Cosmetic Dermatology Associates of Prescott
www.cosmeticdermatologyprescott.com

Expert Advice and Lessons Learned From Some of Today's Most Successful Concierge Medicine, DPC Doctors and Industry Leaders.

Gary Price, MD, FACP
Concierge Physicians Southwest Florida
9722 Commerce Center Court
Fort Myers, FL 33908
Office: 239-415-1111
www.ConciergePhysiciansSWFL.com

Dr. Gary Price writes: "I started my private practice in 1997, I believe one of the first two in the country, the other being Dr. Garrison Bliss and Dr. Howard Maron etc. At that time, nobody had done this, so we didn't have the benefit of "Concierge Medicine Today" or any organization to guide us, so we just invented the wheel and incrementally perfected it until it rolled well."

"The first challenge was opting out of Medicare, which took almost a year to accomplish, as nobody had asked before and they didn't know if there was a mechanism to do it! There was. And now it is a simple process of writing a letter."

"I went through various models, all outside of Medicare and insurance. Initially I did fee-for-service, charging by the visit. Then I experimented with a combination of fee-for-service and retainer (Patients had the option of either model). About 8 years ago I switched to retainer exclusively. My practice has done very well, and about 7 yrs. ago I hired a second physician, whose practice is now about full, so I'm looking for a third doctor."

Brian Thornburg, MSM, DO, PA, FAAP
Innovative Pediatrics
6017 Pine Ridge Road, Suite 148
Naples, FL 34119
Office: 239-348-3563
www.InnovativePediatrics.com
www.ThornburgPediatrics.com

Dr. Brian Thornburg writes: "Thornburg Pediatrics was born out of the usual frustration that arises from the current, traditional medical practice. Insurance hassles with rushed and impersonal care combined with low salary and limited personal time made practicing medicine miserable. I felt there had to be a better way! After spending several years with a large multispecialty group, I decided to focus on wellness, health and prevention. I took a leap of faith, called upon my many years of experience using my Master's degree in business & applied some common sense. With a growing family, I envisioned what I would want in a pediatrician. I developed a practice format around the motto – An Old Fashioned Approach to Modern Medicine™. This is a practice style that allows for great relationships. Parents trust me with the most valuable thing in their lives- their children. Because I am not in a frenzied rush, I am able to practice medicine to the best of my abilities and the difference is incredible."

"I am now my own boss. I maintain an income of twice the national average for pediatricians and have more flexibility for scheduling family and personal time. My overhead is substantially decreased and *I enjoy medicine*. Patients love the practice and tell their friends. I have not had to advertise since my first year of concierge practice. My thoughts for pediatricians considering Concierge Medicine are to believe it can be done. Trust your instincts and do not undersell yourself. You have spent many years learning an incredible depth of knowledge and your vision for a better way to practice exists."

"Since I was the second concierge pediatrician, I had the opportunity to make mistakes and learn what works and what does not. I undersold myself the first year out of fear. This made it difficult to maintain an adequate cash flow and forced me to change my business strategy after the first year. I now charge twice as much per Patient as I did when I started. Educate your community and your Patients. In addition to spending an hour or more at each well child check and about thirty minutes for a sick visit, I hold several lectures a year on various topics including nutrition, environmental health, parenting, discipline and lifestyle. I also coordinate gardening, family yoga, cooking and CPR classes. Additionally, I try to blog daily and send out an e-newsletter two to three times a month. It is important to stay in front of your Patients."

"You should also appreciate professional and personal boundaries. Since you are always available, it is important to learn to say NO. Prioritize and understand the competing needs of family and business. After all, you should be a role model to your families. For example, I try to answer my phone and avoid voicemail after office hours. It is a nice touch to be available and accessible. However your spouse and children need even more respect. When my wife or daughter really needs me, I let the phone call go to voicemail and call the Patient back within minutes. Be mindful that occasionally a Patient's family treats you in an unprofessional manner or abuses the service. Everyone is entitled to a bad day. Watch for patterns of abuse and know that it is okay to discharge families from your practice."

"If you possess excellent communication skills, around the clock dedication and the desire to promote optimal health in pursuit of excellent medicine, then Concierge Medicine is for you. It is the best career choice I have ever made."

"If you possess excellent communication skills, around the clock dedication and the desire to promote optimal health in pursuit of excellent medicine, then Concierge Medicine is for you. It is the best career choice I have ever made."

-Brian Thornburg, MSM, DO, PA, FAAP
Innovative Pediatrics
www.InnovativePediatrics.com
www.ThornburgPediatrics.com

Chapter 8 –
Your Journey Begins Now.

Retirement Planning: Sell-Out or A Slow Burn.

We all think about it, especially when the average age of most Concierge Doctors is 55+ years of age, according to *Concierge Medicine Today*. Medical analysts and healthcare thought leaders predict that 2015 will be a record breaking year in terms of doctors selling their practices, merging with hospitals and specialty clinics and physicians retiring. According to Deloitte's 2013 Survey of U.S. Physicians, it is estimated that fifty percent of doctors will work for a hospital-owned or affiliated medical center group or health system of some kind.

For many physicians approaching retirement, one of the following paths is usually taken:

- **Selling Your Practice** – Preparing a valuation of the practice and choosing to select a younger doctor(s) to handle Patient care. Helping to ease this transition for Patients, most retiring physicians allow the new doctor to shadow their movements, make introductions and eventually, phase out of the practice operations entirely;
- **The Slow Burn** – Working a few hours a week or every month just to stay active. Never really retiring, but allowing yourself to stay engaged in medicine;

Investors tell *Concierge Medicine Today* that most Concierge Medicine practices can be worth at most, between four and five times the net profit after the physician is paid as an employee, sometimes called a cap rate or capitalization rate method of placing a value on the practice.

Patients (i.e. members or subscribers) are considered strong, valuable assets in any business preparing to sell. When it is time to retire, bringing on a younger (not too young), doctor to shadow you for a year is the wisest approach according to some industry consultants. Because most Patients/Members have contracts with the practice and not the doctor him/herself for legal purposes, these members are property of the practice, so-to-speak, and bring enormous value to the practice.

"The key to success in any Concierge Medicine or DPC practice is, and always will be, the relationship that the doctor has with his or her Patients," notes Mike Permenter, industry Consultant. "With that in mind, one of the most important things for a new or established doctor to do is to constantly strive to improve the value proposition — at the Patient level. The more you can do to improve the Patient experience, the better each doctor's financial returns are likely to be. Successful doctors need less in the way of support after the operational and internal planning has been done and should be hesitant to sign long-term contracts for longer than three or five years. Of course, a long-term contract can bring more Patients and make your practice more profitable, thus improving the eventual sale of your practice or retirement plan. Nothing sells a concierge medical practice faster than Patients that are exuberant about their experiences with a particular doctor's office."

Hybrid Concierge Medicine clinics are by far the most popular according to industry analyses. More often than not, these types of medical business models retain more Patients inside the practice database because they continue to accept and participate in most insurance plans and offer membership packages as an added value program.

For those doctors looking for ways to retire, remain financially independent of hospital-owned systems or are still years away from retirement, the probability of eventually selling your Concierge Medicine practice for a profit is highly likely.

For younger physicians looking for a career in this industry, shadowing a retiring physician for a couple of years offers a unique alternative to starting your own concierge practice from scratch or working for the local hospital system. It has been touted that full Hybrid Concierge programs are generally more profitable than traditional, managed care and insurance-based medical practices because they bring value to both the seller and buyer. Why? This is due in part to primary care practices with concierge programs as added value add-ons in place plus the ability to acquire Patients through HMO, PPO and POS networks has assurances that their investment is more secure.

As Concierge Medicine and DPC grows in use and popularity, more HR Managers, benefit administrators, self-insured business owners and larger employer organizations are going to recognize the value it can bring to an employee population. We believe that in the next ten years, we will begin to see more and more primary care and family medical doctors partnering with self-insured businesses and employer groups to provide healthcare programs that serve a unique workplace health need.

For more resources, individuals and attorneys that can assist you in your business planning and retirement assistance, visit www.ConciergeMedicineToday.com.

"The field of Concierge Medicine and DPC (DPC) is still relatively young but the ideology pre-dates the telephone and even the Revolutionary War ... whereby a doctor comes to your aid, day or night, there is no-copay, deductible or appointment required," says Michael Tetreault, Editor of Concierge Medicine Today. "Concierge Medicine physicians and DPC doctors stand in the gap for you. They are reducing hospitalizations significantly, compatible with nearly every insurance plan in America and people are saving more money on their healthcare costs each year. More people are enrolling in high-deductible health insurance plans that cover major, unforeseen events, leaving the everyday expenses to the consumer—just like auto and homeowners' insurance."

"I knew I was being compromised by seeing Patients every eight to 10 minutes just to keep the doors open,"

-Dr. Jack Padour, Ventura, CALIF.

Moving The Needle Forward.

What is next for the future of Concierge Medicine, DPC clinics, direct pay practices, retail medicine and convenient care clinics? We believe that the more doctors (not office managers, staff or nurses), communicate with Patients face-to-face and provide other value-driven options, the more those Patients will come back again and again. Better yet, they will tell their friends and family to see you too. After all, what primary care or family medical practice do you know of today that spends more than 45 to 90 minutes with each Patient on every visit?

In surveying thousands of physicians for the nonprofit Physicians Foundation, Merritt Hawkins, a national consulting and search firm in Irving, Texas, recently reported that about 7% of respondents said they were planning to transition to concierge or cash-only practices in the next one to three years.

At *Concierge Medicine Today*, we believe the growth rate will be much higher in the coming years – possibly around 15% due to the Affordable Care Act (ACA). Although this is our opinion, we have certainly seen an increase in physician interest to support it.

Overall, Concierge Medicine, boutique healthcare, DPC or whatever you would like to name it is thriving in major metropolitan markets. Prices are dropping dramatically due to increasing competition among physicians entering the marketplace, retail medicine pricing, price transparency demand from Patients and uncertainty about the implications of the Affordable Care Act.

Proposed Industry Guidelines

As we conclude this Guidebook, we thought it wise and important to summarize and filter through the conclusions that many in the industry have written over the years. While the AMA and AAFP have written and developed a foundational base upon which to create industry guidelines, nothing formal has to this date been followed or abided by in the Concierge Medicine or DPC industry.

No Accountable Care Organizations (ACO) have been created to our knowledge, although at Concierge Medicine Today, we have discussed the creation of this type of governing or credentialing body in-depth with industry influencers. As the years go by, we are certain that the debate will most likely continue and it should. Experts in this industry conclude the following:

- A Patient must be familiar with Concierge Care and DPC and understand the contract in which they are about to enter into with the doctor. Each Patient should conduct their own research both pertaining to the Physician they select and the contract they sign. They should be aware of what services are covered by their insurance versus the concierge retainer agreement.

- The Physician must examine his/her motivation for switching to Concierge Medicine or DPC. Concierge physicians tend to have less insurance paperwork to file, less support staff and fewer total Patients.
- Experts, writers, doctors and attorneys do not feel that the United States government should have the authority to determine whether or not direct-pay, DPC, Concierge or membership medicine style practice models can operate, like in Canada. Physicians should have the right to choose which customers (i.e. Patients) they serve.
- Many physicians find that they are dissatisfied with their own work and the quality of care that their Patients are receiving because of the lack of time and appropriate compensation. Switching to a Concierge Medicine or DPC membership-based medical practice based on the best interests of their Patients is not only admirable, but strongly encouraged by those inside and outside of the healthcare industry.
- It is advised that services offered in a Concierge or DPC practice should medically contribute to the well-being of the Patient. It is not recommended that excessive and extravagant services that have little to no medical value.
- Experts, writers, doctors and attorney's recommend that Concierge Medicine and DPC physicians set up a separate business corporation alongside their professional corporation if they choose to bill insurers. These types of Physicians should distinguish between the covered services for which they are collecting a fee, and the uncovered services for which they are billing insurance. Physicians are encouraged to develop a "menu" of fees and services to offer.
- The issue of Patient abandonment is of great concern when Concierge Medicine and DPC is discussed in the marketplace. The Physician making the switch to Concierge Medicine should keep the Patients that they will lose in highest priority, making sure the appropriate arrangements are made to find them a new Physician. If a Physician chooses to transition and/or start a Concierge or DPC medical or membership practice, there will be hundreds of Patients searching for a new Physician. Each transitioning physician should assist those Patients not enrolling into the program and help them have a smooth transition to their new doctor. This will provide the best continuity of care for Patients.
- Experts, writers, doctors and attorney's recommend that younger, newer physicians consider Concierge Medicine and DPC although it is more difficult to enter as a startup because there is no existing Patient base upon which to draw. As a new physician, it is very difficult to start a Concierge Medicine or DPC medical practice right from residency, but it is possible if joining an existing practice.
- Experts, writers, doctors and attorney's believe that a concierge practice should offer scholarships that would address the needs of minorities, the poor, the elderly and those unable to afford insurance. This would help to eliminate any disparities in healthcare. Physicians should make their services accessible to all Patients, giving back to the community in which they serve.

At *Concierge Medicine Today*, we believe this form of healthcare and other forms including: retail medicine; retainer medicine; cash-only healthcare; DPC; direct care; boutique medicine; etc., be treated seriously by insurers, hospitals, physicians and Patients alike. It is a concept that is here to stay. Paying a set fee for "non-covered services" may appear to some to focus on money or greed but to the majority of the American population, it redirects the focus of medicine back to preventing disease and seeking wellness. It is the way medicine and healthcare used to be before the 1960's and government regulation. If concierge, DPC and retainer medicine doctors are successful in preventing illness, which data and studies are beginning to show and are helping to keep Patients healthier longer, it is in the best interest of insurers, business leaders, legislators, Patients, and society as a whole to encourage its growth.

Six Traits Great Concierge Medicine and DPC Doctors Share.

To conclude this book, we asked some of the industry's leading physicians and business owners, 'What are the traits of a Concierge Doctor or DPC physician business owner?'

From the onset, the idea of starting or even moving your medical practice into this marketplace seems inspiring, but also intimidating. Scholars, physicians, business experts and venture capitalists say Concierge Medicine and DPC is a growing industry. But, as we have learned over the years, the best Concierge and DPC Doctors share a collection of characteristics, from the ability to tolerate risk, treating 5 to 9 Patients per day, risking reputation over reward to passion and self-belief in a niche-industry.

1. Tenacity.

Physicians explained this process as a marathon, not a race. More of an ultra-marathon really, dependent upon which individuals you might talk with. Nonetheless, you have to be able to live with uncertainty and push through a crucible of challenges and obstacles for a couple of years.

"I received a phone call the other day from a physician in Winter Park Florida," says Tiffany Sizemore-Ruiz, D.O. of Choice Physicians of South Florida. "She was calling just to thank me for answering her questions about Concierge Medicine a few months ago, and encouraging her to start her own concierge practice. Today, her practice is thriving and she said that 'she is happy with her schedule, her life, and being able to practice medicine that way it is meant to be practiced.' I was so happy to hear that I helped a fellow physician and colleague, and even more happy to hear that she was doing so well!"

"The conversion process is not an easy one," said Jeffrey S. Gorodetsky, M.D. of Stuart, FL. "My staff and I are cognizant of the fact that we must consistently communicate the benefits of this choice in care, with the challenge to increase my concierge numbers and convert my non-concierge Patients."

2. Passion.

"If you possess excellent communication skills, around the clock dedication and the desire to promote optimal health in pursuit of excellent medicine, then Concierge Medicine is for you. It is the best career choice I have ever made," says Brian Thornburg, MSM, DO, PA, and FAAP of Innovative Pediatrics.

Second, it is commonly presumed that doctors who enter Concierge Medicine are driven to do so by money. What most doctors who have been there and done that will tell you is ... 'I'm fueled by a passion to help my Patients. I'm now allowed the opportunity to problem-solve and make life a little easier, better and cheaper for my Patients.'

3. Managing Fear, Uncertainty and Potential Failure.

"The doctor of the future will no longer treat the human frame with drugs, but rather will cure and prevent disease with nutrition." ~Thomas Edison

The ability to successfully manage fear. Risk-taking goes with the territory when you talk about Concierge Medicine with most physicians, consultants and staff. 'I do not think my Patients are going to like this,' most say. But your ability to withstand the pressure and overcome the obstacles of uncertainty and potential failure and see the other side before others do is what makes a successful Concierge Physician, notes one industry consultant. He sees that the ability for doctors to control their doubt and fear as the most important trait of all.

4. Vision and Task-Specific Confidence.

"In selecting only a small population of clients and providing dedicated counseling sessions, sometimes as often as weekly, allows clients to actively participate in their care plan and to move goals forward at a real-time pace. This enables all of us to realize that healthcare can be a positive experience," notes Dr. Carrie Bordinko of Consolaré Primary Care in Paradise Valley, AZ

Physicians who have traveled down this path over the past 15 years imagine another world free from insurance burdens and heavy administrative overhead. They envision spending more time with Patients and enjoying the practice of medicine again. Oftentimes, these physicians and medical practice business owners will find themselves facing naysayers, says one doctor in New York. 'We often see the future before it plays out. We have to be prepared to be several steps ahead of the market.'

If you have planned appropriately, conducted enough analysis and have sufficient research that you can provide the level of service you envision for your medical practice's future to ameliorate the risk, you are ready to take the next step.

"I remember when I started my direct-access, home-based primary care practice (www.MetroMedicalDirect.com) in 2009," says Raymond Zakhari, NP and CEO of Metro Medical Direct. "Patients were skeptical and reluctant because of how accessible and convenient the service was. They expected to be kept waiting on hold. Some seemed puzzled by the fact that when they called I answered the phone and knew who they were. One Patient even inquired as to how come they only had one form to fill out. Direct-access primary care Patients who have been referred post hospital discharge, have not been readmitted to the hospital in the last 4 years because I can see them without delay or red tape. In NYC, despite the high number

356

of physicians per Patient, particularly on the upper east side of Manhattan, direct-access primary care can still be a viable practice solution for Patients and providers. It helps Patients cut through the red tape that has become expected in accessing health care."

5. Planning, Flexibility.

It is likely that your final service or product offering will not look anything like that with which you started. Planning ahead, being flexible and your willingness to defy conventional wisdom will help you respond to changes in the economy, insurance and market forces that seem to dislike your current operation. You have to be able to pivot when necessary.

"One of the most difficult occurrences is when Patients who do not understand the program or who philosophically disagrees with the membership fees (i.e. thinks this is for rich people) accuse the physician of abandoning them," says one former Transition Manager in Arizona. "Sometimes Patients can be very vocal about their opinion on this and at times, be quite rude. This is very disheartening to most doctors, at least in the early stages of the transition process. 'Saying goodbye' to some long-term Patients is one of the reasons many Physicians are reluctant to convert."

6. Rule-Breaking.

"Instead of viewing the status quo PCP model as the center of the universe. Maybe we should take some plays from the Retail Clinic playbook before we become obsolete," not DPC physician, Dr. Robert Nelson of Cumming, GA.

Even the thought of starting a Concierge Medicine or DPC medical practice or program in your local community defies conventional wisdom according to many people in the healthcare marketplace. If you consider the fact that 13 percent of Americans are engaged in start-up businesses, according to a Babson College report, doing what the majority of doctors are doing nowadays is not in your future. You are a risk-taker.

Are these characteristics or traits in you? There is only one way to find out.

Seek Expert Advice, Guidance and Resources.

At *Concierge Medicine Today*, we focus on reporting and writing the news — not to sell you someone or something. You should choose who you work with — but you should choose wisely. Here's where you start. By popular demand, we have assembled and added specific categories to help doctors, business-owners and individuals connect with trusted, ethical, relational and knowledgeable experts in the Concierge Medicine and DPC marketplace that you can trust and we have thoroughly examined. Visit www.ConciergeMedicineToday.com to learn more.

"Please do not go it alone....seek advice/guidance with those of us that have experience. Make sure you understand the medical legal aspects of this that might be very specific for your state."

-Joel Bessmer, MD, FACP, Omaha, NE

"I use a PayPal merchant account to process cards."
-Dr. Marina Gafanovich MD, New York, NY

Chapter 9 – Supportive Resources.

All referral agents recommended to you by "Concierge Medicine Today," The "Direct Primary Care Journal" or "The Collective" are independent agents with the ability to perform their service(s). All recommended agents are licensed in their respective states to perform specific business services and as we understand, are in accordance with their State laws. All questions or problems that arise with regard to any transaction should be sent to the referred agent. For more information, please contact our office at 770-455-1650.

"The Collective," "The Direct Primary Care Journal" and/or "Concierge Medicine Today" is not in the business of offering any type of legal or financial information regarding your specific situation. These matters are to be handled solely by the "agents" or recommended professionals you select. We are not responsible in any way for the actions of these individuals or companies, monetarily or otherwise, and you understand that these recommended resources and connections may use your personal information to contact you and to better serve you.

Legal Notice And Disclaimer

This book, articles, web site(s), programs and all other associated reference guides and materials are designed to provide accurate and authoritative information with regard to the subject matter covered. The information is given with the understanding that the authors, publishers, distributors, publisher, its related, affiliated or subsidiary companies, are not engaging in or rendering legal, accounting or other professional advice. The authors, publishers, distributors, publisher, its related, affiliated or subsidiary companies, stress that since the details of an individual's personal situation are fact-dependent, you should seek the additional services of a competent professional.

It is your responsibility to evaluate the accuracy, completeness and usefulness of any opinions, advice, services or other information provided. All information contained on any page of this or other affiliated works is distributed with the understanding that the authors, publishers, distributors publisher, its related, affiliated or subsidiary companies, are not rendering legal, accounting or other professional advice or opinions on specific facts or matters, and accordingly, assume no liability whatsoever in connection with its use. Consult your own legal or tax advisor with respect to your personal situation.

In no event shall the authors, publishers, distributors publisher, its related, affiliated or subsidiary companies, be liable for any direct, indirect, special, incidental or consequential damages arising out of the use of the information herein.

Expert Advice, Guidance and Resources. Safe, Secure and Trusted.
Our "Endorsed Industry Service Provider" (or EIP) Panel Is NOT Bought — It is Earned.

Our focus at *Concierge Medicine Today* is on reporting and writing the news — not to sell you services or individuals. You should choose who you work with — but you should choose wisely. Here's where you start. By popular demand, we have assembled and added categories (See Below) to help doctors, business-owners and individuals connect with trusted, ethical, relational and knowledgeable experts in the Concierge Medicine and DPC marketplace that people can trust and we have examined.

We have found the brightest Concierge Medicine and DPC marketplace's top-notch individuals, leaders and companies to help you in your practice — no matter what phase you are in. *Concierge Medicine Today's* Innovators Panel is not bought – it is earned. We partner only with individuals and companies who hold themselves to a higher standard of excellence, have a proven track-record in the Concierge Medicine and DPC space and are passionate about making things happen and bringing ideas to execution for doctors and staff. In many ways, innovation is key to your success no matter in what phase of development your practice is currently in. The minute you stop innovating is the minute you become mediocre.

Typically, Our EIP Panel Falls Into One of 3 Categories:

- **Startup Experts** ... with experience in multiple startups.
- **Industry Experts** ... individuals with a wealth of industry-specific experience.
- **Knowledge Experts** ... mentors with experience in a specific range of business skills (Legal, Accounting, Finance, Marketing, IT, Infrastructure, Operations, etc...)

You will be amazed by the level of advice and customer service our EIP (Endorsed Industry Service Provider) Panel provides to physicians, Patients and businesses. Our network of Concierge Medicine and DPC companies, businesses, mentors and coaches can discuss with you your needs and provide nonbiased information and guidance you can trust. They will give you sound guidance — without any sales pitch.

Simply drop us a line or send us an email to Editor@conciergemedicinetoday.com and we'll review your inquiry and send you the contact information for the EIP (Endorsed Industry Service Provider) Panel Member in your area!

Until recently, people mostly based choosing a doctor on the personal recommendation of a trusted friend or relative. Now with the advent of social media, word of mouth marketing is changing from a spoken word referral to a social media link referral. To find a Concierge Medicine or direct care doctor near you, Concierge Medicine Today has created an iTunes and Android App, Concierge Doc, a free App and search engine resource to find and learn about Concierge Medicine and DPC in your area is available at ConciergeMedicineToday.com.

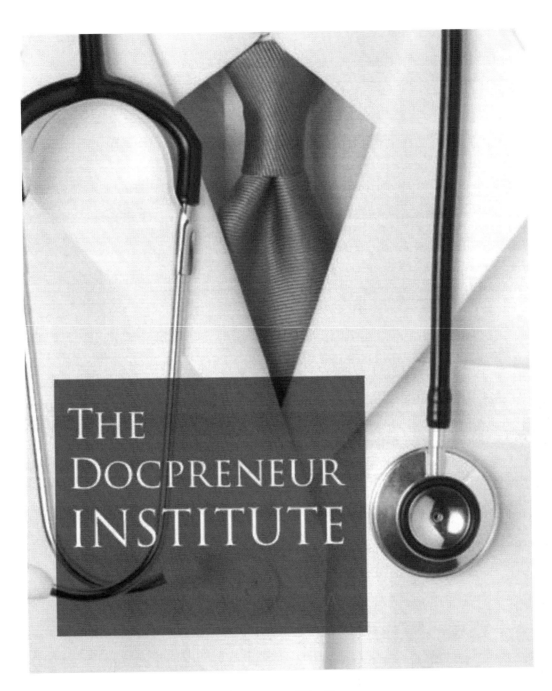

Learn More, visit www.TheDocpreneur.org

Startups & Strategy: Mentors & Coaches

for the Docpreneur in you ...

In Partnership with The Docpreneur Insititute © 2015

Effective and affordable, and you only pay for the time you need. Our coaches specialize in providing solutions without an annoying sales pitch.

Learn More, visit www.TheDocpreneur.org

DPC Mentor &
Coaching
for the Docpreneur in you ...

In Partnership with The Docpreneur Insititute © 2015

Effective and affordable, and you only pay for the time you need. Our coaches specialize in providing solutions without an annoying sales pitch.

Learn More, visit www.TheDocpreneur.org

Public Resources: INDUSTRY NEWS AND INFORMATION
Concierge Medicine Today

Concierge Medicine Today (CMT), is the premier news and multi-media organization and the industry's oldest national trade publication for the DPC and Concierge Medicine marketplace. Their web site is the online destination for business, consumers and physicians to learn about the history of this industry, various business aspects of the marketplace, trends, breaking news and more that drive the conversation and generate the national buzz that Concierge Medicine and DPC is creating on a national and international level. For more information, visit: http://www.ConciergeMedicineToday.com or call tel: 770-455-1650.

RESEARCH, STATS, NUMBERS and MORE!
The Concierge Medicine Research Collective

The Concierge Medicine Research Collective is a research and data depository created by Concierge Medicine Today. The Concierge Medicine Research Collective is an independent health care research and data collection depository of the multimedia news and trade publication, Concierge Medicine Today based in Atlanta, GA. The Collective serves as an educational resource on all things Concierge Medicine and is geared towards those businesses, lobbyists, physician associations, health care advocacy groups and general consumers of healthcare who want to learn more about information available on the topic of Concierge Medicine.

The Collective works in partnership with Universities, physicians, institutions, associations, businesses, individuals and medical schools to further advance the educational awareness and facts surrounding unanswered questions about Concierge Medicine care in the U.S. and Canada. For more information, visit: http://www.AskTheCollective.org or call tel: 770-455-1650.

INDUSTRY NEWS AND INFORMATION
The DPC Journal

The Direct Primary Care Journal (DPC Journal) is an independent online news reporting publication and trade journal utilizing journalists and dedicated writers who cover all facets of the DPC [direct care] industry. For more information, news or to locate a DPC doctor, visit: www.DirectCareJournal.com or www.DirectPrimaryCare.com or call tel: 770-455-1650.

The Docpreneur Institute (DPI)
DISTANCE LEARNING | BUSINESS EDUCATION and PHYSICIAN
MENTOR/COACHING

In 2014, *Concierge Medicine Today* launched The Docpreneur Institute (DPI), a partnership of local and national industry business leaders, private interests and the concierge physician community at-large with the mission to raise the quality of resources available to the entrepreneurial physician and small business community and create businesses and connecting them with quality resources and people to network with and be mentored by. *Concierge Medicine Today* and *The Direct Primary Care Journal* have become became the front door for countless physician entrepreneurs. Their Docpreneur Institute connects physician-entrepreneurs with accomplished professionals [and experienced physician mentors] you can learn from — pros who give the same helpful advice that so thousands of people read about in our publications every day. CMTs Docpreneur Institute "Mentor Meetings" are limited to ten (10) physicians each month and available by application only beginning in January of 2015.

The Docpreneur Institute (DPI) was launched to give physicians access to objective and experienced mentors who can answer their questions, provide feedback, insight and guidance as they evaluate starting a medical practice, growing a local clinic, hiring staff, marketing, learning about starting a concierge medicine or Direct Primary Care (DPC) model, or determining which business relationships your practice should have with payors. For more information, visit: www.TheDocpreneur.org.

HOW TO LOCATE A CONCIERGE DOCTOR OR DIRECT PAY PHYSICIAN

Until recently, people mostly based choosing a doctor on the personal recommendation of a trusted friend or relative. Now with the advent of social media, word of mouth marketing is changing from a spoken word referral to a social media link referral. To find a Concierge Medicine or DPC doctor near you, Concierge Medicine Today has created an iTunes and Android App, Concierge Doc, a free App and search engine resource to find and learn about Concierge Medicine and DPC in your area. It is available at ConciergeMedicineToday.com.

If you'd like to find a medical home, Concierge Physician or DPC physician in your area or simply to learn more about them, you will want to visit: www.ConciergeMedicineToday.com or www.DirectPrimaryCare.com. If you are unable to locate one using these national directories, we recommend you call Concierge Medicine Today at 770-455-1650 and a representative will be happy to help you.

Recommended Reading

Concierge Medicine Today Launches "Legal Center," a Digital Library and Resource For Physicians and Businesses Considering a Career In Concierge Medicine or DPC –

Concierge Medicine Today's "Legal Center" will serve as the industry's central digital library for reports, letters, opinions, legal news, important information, and policy happenings for doctors, venture capitalists and business leaders considering a career or future endeavor in this marketplace.

Available at: www.ConciergeMedicineToday.com

Direct Primary Care Journal releases Third Edition of "DPC Consumer/Patient Guide."

JANUARY 15, 2015 | ATLANTA, GA USA - The Direct Primary Care Journal (DPC Journal) is starting the New Year with the release of the Print and Kindle Edition of its "*Direct Primary Care (DPC) Consumer Guide*" which includes more than 60 new or updated entries, broadens the FAQs asked by people finding a doctor and defines with greater clarity the Direct Primary Care service offering being delivered by doctors and clinics throughout the U.S. in 2015.

At about 98+ pages, "*The DPC Consumer Guide*" is widely used in physician offices. undergraduate and medical college classrooms, and corporate offices worldwide. More than a dozen of the new entries in the 2015 Edition are in the sections on FAQs About DPC, which include: The Difference Between Concierge Medicine and Direct Primary Care (DPC); How Does This Work With My Flex Spending Account, Medical Savings, HSA or HRA? and Does DPC pair well with insurance plans? and more.

The definition entries have been updated and consolidated for easier understanding. The 50-Point Checklist of 'Must Ask Questions To Ask A DPC Doctor Before You Sign-Up' provides a useful reference for anyone interviewing their next direct-pay primary care doctor's office.

The new definition entries on the difference between Concierge Medicine and Direct Primary Care give readers helpful guidelines on the cost, services and insurance component variances associated with the two different sectors within Membership Medicine healthcare in America today. The glossary entry defining the "Membership Medicine" classification, a term widely used by investment and private equity firms when talking about Direct Primary Care, is also added to the book to provide further understanding and clarification of the various types of clinics now available to people.

The 3rd Edition of "*The DPC Consumer Guide: 2015 Edition*" consolidates a number of changes made since the first volume, published by *The DPC Journal*.

"Updated annually since its initial publication in 2012, the *DPC Consumer Guide* is a must-have reference for doctors, patients, students and medical professionals," says Michael Tetreault, Editor and co-author of the book. "It provides fundamental educational information about a growing healthcare sector and it is the definitive resource for people wanting to learn more about Direct Primary Care and can benefit their wallet and their family."

The new print edition can be ordered online at www.DirectPrimarCare.org and is sold also on Amazon, Barnes and Noble and other online book retailers.

The new paperback "DPC Consumer Guide: 2015 Edition" costs $8.95 for and $11.95 retail. Bulk orders for classrooms, doctors' offices and events are available in minimum orders of 25-50.

Email or contact The DPC Journal Bookstore for a list of bulk order prices. Prices for the Kindle version of the book are $5.95. Education Institutions and non-profits may also receive discounts. Email editor@directcarejournal.com or call 770-455-1650 to inquire.

About The Direct Primary Care Journal

The Direct Primary Care Journal (The DPC Journal) is an independent trade journal and multimedia news reporting publication observing, reporting, resourcing and connecting with experts from all facets of the DPC industry. For more information, visit: DirectPrimaryCare.org.

Sited Sources –

- [1] For more on the Thompson letter and its historical context, see the author's article: "Legal Issues Involved in Concierge Medical Practices," www.wnj.com/concierge_practices_jrm_3_2005/.
- [2] One blogger suggested that there are about 5,000 concierge physicians operating in the United States. http://www.managemypractice.com. He does not cite his source for this, but the suggestion is most certainly inflated, by a lot. The authors of a March of 2010, MedPAC report ("Retainer-Based Physicians: Characteristics, Impact, and Policy Considerations") (see www.medpac.gov) could find fewer than 800 such practices, although they acknowledged that their number would likely be the lower limit of the actual one.
- [3] Public Law No. 111-148, March 10, 2010.
- [4] Patients around that time had complained that physicians converting their practices to the FNCS concierge model were requiring them to pay an annual lump-sum fee or find another physician.
- [5] There is also an issue whether FNCS practices square with the provisions of private contracts between physicians and insurance companies. These issues are not uniform from insurance company to insurance company and are not, in terms of their effect on physicians, as daunting as those presented by Medicare.
- [6] See the author's article *The Politics of Concierge Medicine; the Vulnerability of the FNCS Model*, www.wnj.com/politics_of_concierge_medicine_jrm_article/) for a more in-depth treatment of the Fraud Alert.
- [7] The physician agreed to waive the Patient's co-pays in exchange for the annual fee.
- [8] See Charles B. Root, "New Medicare Preventive Services and Screening Tests You Can Perform in the Office," *Medicare Patient Management*, March/April 2006, page18, http://www.medicare Patientmanagement.com/issues/01-02/MPM01-02_Screening.pdf.
- [9] The technical name for this physical exam is the Initial Preventive Physical Exam. See 42 USC 1395x(ww).
- [10] This led some physicians to postpone any physical exam for a new Medicare Patient until AFTER the six months of her Medicare coverage expired to ensure that the physical exam could not possibly be mistaken for the IPPE. Aside from the obvious ethical problems with this approach, as a practical matter this shenanigan was put to rest in 2007 when the eligibility for the IPPE was extended to the full year of a Patient's Medicare coverage.
- [11] There are no co-pays or deductibles associated with the AWV. Medicare pays 100%.
- [12] http://oig.hhs.gov/fraud/physicianeducation.
- [13] See the author's article "Suggested Modifications to Fee for Non-Covered Services Concierge Practices as a Result of New Healthcare Act," http://www.wnj.com/suggested_modifications_to_fee_for_non-covered_services_concierge_practices_as_a_result_of_non_health_care_act-concierge_law/.
- [14] 75 Fed Register 73170-01, November 29, 2010.
- [15] Some services listed would not be covered in an annual wellness context, at least every year, but some would be covered even in a wellness context in certain years and as part of a physical if medically indicated as part of an underlying diagnosis. A screening EKG, for instance, is covered by Medicare on a one-time basis, but an EKG is also covered in a non-screening context if indicated as part of a diagnosis and is medically indicated.
- [16] Some anti-Concierge Medicine public officials, like the New Jersey and New York health departments (for copies of the letters from these departments see www.wnj.com/practiceindustries/retainermed/legal_developments/), have suggested that physicians already, as a matter of course, give or are obligated to give their Patients 24/7 access. Such a suggestion reveals a bias that is not supported by any real analysis or even much awareness. Very few non-concierge physicians expose themselves, personally, to 24/7 direct contact by Patients. Certainly Patients of most primary care physicians can "reach" their physician 24/7 by called an answering service, which then routes the Patients to a covering physician, and maybe directly to the Patients' actual physician if he or she happens to be on call. But that is much different than the Patient paying the concierge physician a special fee in order to have direct 24/7 access to her physician at all times.
- [17] Nothing in this comment should be taken as legal advice. Any physician contemplating including one or more of these services in a Patient agreement should consult his or her attorney.

- [18]Another reason this result will be disappointing to many concierge physicians is its effect on efforts to inform Patients that the special fee is an expense that can be paid from a Health Savings Account, another so-called "acronym plan" (like an FSA and MSA), or a cafeteria plan. Concierge physicians are notorious for jumping to conclusions as to the applicability of these plans to special Concierge Medicine fees. But this entire area is cloudy and uncertain and no one can be sure, under existing law, whether any part of a concierge fee can qualify for any of them. However, the chances they can qualify increase if the special fee is paid for medical care, like an annual physical. If only "amenities" are included in the special fee, then there is likely no chance the payments will qualify. A similar point can be made about whether the special fee can count toward a Patient's deductible amount under a high-deductible health insurance policy.

- [19]And there are others that would not likely trigger a Medicare problem because they are not medical services. For instance, some physicians include "friends and family" provision that allows friends and family visiting or vacationing with the concierge Patient to have the same direct access to the physician for a limited number of days during the year.

- [20]Recall in footnote 12 the reference to the new CMS publication warning new physicians that charging an "'access fee' or 'administrative fee' that simply allows them to obtain Medicare-covered services from your practice" amounts to double billing. This reference to an "access" or "administrative" fee should not be taken as referring to providing the Patient with something special that has value in the market place, like personal, direct, 24/7 coverage or friends and family access, things that a physician is not otherwise obligated (legally or ethically) to do for Patients. The reference should be taken to mean those sorts of across-the-board charges that are little more than surcharges to Patients just so they can continue to belong to a practice. There have been reports of physicians billing all their Patients a small amount annually to help the physician with his or her overhead. Such charges are without much question illegal.

- Gottschalk A, Flocke SA. Time spent in face-to-face Patient care and work outside the examination room. Ann Fam Med.2005;3(6):488-493.

- Ii. Solomon J. How strategies for managing Patient visit time affect physician job satisfaction: a qualitative analysis. J Gen Intern Med. 2008;23(6):775-780.

- Iii. American Academy of Family Physicians. Teamwork within a practice can relieve Patient overload. AAFP News Now. October 9, 2012. www.aafp.org/online/en/home/publications/news/news-now/practice-professional-issues/20121009teambasedcare.html.

- Iv. Murray M, Davies M, Boushon B. Panel size: how many Patients can one doctor manage?

- FPM. 2007:14(4):44-51.

- V. Kong MC, Camacho FT, Feldman SR, Anderson RT, Balkrishnan R. Correlates of Patient satisfaction with physician visit: differences between elderly and non-elderly survey respondents.

- Health and Quality of Life Outcomes. 2007;5(62). www.hqlo.com/content/5/1/62.

- Vi. Dugdale DC, Epstein R, Pantilat SZ. Time and the Patient–physician relationship. J Gen Intern Med.1999:14(S)S34-S40.

- Vii. Wasson JH, Anders SG, Moore LG, Ho L, Nelson EC, Godfrey MM, et al. Clinical microsystems, art 2. Learning from micro practices about providing Patients the care they want and need. The Joint Commission Journal on Quality and Patient Safety. 2008:34(8):445-452

- http://host.madison.com/news/local/writers/steven_elbow/affordable-concierge-medicine-doc-closes-up-shop/article_53513f32-a6f8-5336-86a0-dc24c5804e8b.html#ixzz2lNlHrVmZ

- How much does it cost to run a concierge medical practice?http://atlas.md/blog/2013/06/how-much-does-it-cost-to-run-a-concierge-medical-practice/#more-640

- With contributions by Mike Permenter, CMT Contributing Writer

- Roberta Greenspan of Specialdocs

- Richard Doughty of Cypress Concierge Medicine

- Scott Borden of Direct Pay Consulting

- Dr. Chris Ewin of 121MD in Fort Worth, TX

- http://www.caringtoday.com/manage-medications/the-importance-of-medication-compliance

- http://www.AskTheCollective.org

- http://www.conciergemedicinetoday.com/

- The Physicians Foundation. A survey of America's physicians: practice patterns and perspectives. September 2012. http://www.physiciansfoundation.org/uploads/default/Physicians_Foundation_2012_Biennial_Survey.pdf Accessed April 23, 2014.

- Association of American Medical Colleges. 2013 state physician workforce data book. November 2013. https://www.aamc.org/download/362168/data/2013statephysicianworkforcedatabook.pdf Accessed April 24, 2014.

- http://directprimarycarejournal.com/2014/05/19/medscapewebmd-cash-only-practices-8-issues-to-consider/

- Medscape Business of Medicine © 2014 WebMD, LLC; http://www.medscape.com/viewarticle/824543_1

- Article Citation: Cash-Only Practices: 8 Issues to Consider. *Medscape*. May 15, 2014.

- http://theadvocate.com/news/business/6242079-123/converting-to-concierge

- Carnahan, S. J. (2007, Spring). Concierge medicine: Legal and ethical issues. *The Journal of Law, Medicine, and Ethics, 35*(1), 211-215.

- The Concierge Medicine Research Collective [The Collective]. (2013). Concierge medicine cost. *Concierge Medicine Today: Concierge Medicine News*. Retrieved from http://conciergemedicinenews.wordpress.com/concierge-medicine-cost/

- Concierge Medicine Today [CMT]. (2013, November). *Concierge medicine doctor infographic*. Retrieved from http://conciergemedicinenews.files.wordpress.com/2013/11/concierge-medicine-doctor-infographic-2014.jpg

- Concierge Medicine Today [CMT]. (2014a, April). *Concierge medicine: 101*. C. Sykes & M. Tetreault (Eds.), 1-28. Retrieved from http://conciergemedicinenews.files.wordpress.com/2014/04/concierge-medicine-101.pdf

- Concierge Medicine Today [CMT]. (2014b, May 19). *2014 Concierge physician salary report*. Retrieved from http://conciergemedicinenews.wordpress.com/2014-concierge-physician-salary-report/

- McDonough, S. (2013, February 5). Paying for an open medical door. *Canadian Medical Association Journal, 185*(2), E105-E106. doi: 10.1503/cmaj.109-4385

- Miscoe, M. D. (2006). Is your marketing compliant? Federal regulations dictate what you can and cannot do to attract patients. *Chiropractic Economics*. Retrieved from http://www.chiroeco.com/article/2006/Issue1/Legl.php

- Press, M. J. (2011). Improvement happens: An interview with Deeb Salem, MD and Brian Cohen, MD. *Journal of General Internal Medicine, 27*(3), 381-385. doi: 10.1007/s11606-011-1947-7

- Tetreault, M. (2014, February 20). Concierge medicine's best kept secret, the price (revised). *Concierge Medicine Today and Direct Primary Care Journal*. Retrieved from http://conciergemedicinenews.wordpress.com/2014/02/20/concierge-medicines-best-kept-secret-the-price-revised/

- Wieczner, J. (2013, November 10). Pros and cons of concierge medicine: More practices are catering to the middle class, with the goal of providing affordable care. *Wall Street Journal*. Retrieved from http://search.proquest.com/docview/1449678285?accountid=458

- http://amac.us/concierge-medicine-alternative-insurance/

- http://www.henrycountytimes.com/Archives/2013/03.27.13/feature.htm

- http://www.americantelemed.org/about-telemedicine/what-is-telemedicine#.VNpSES6fUUM

- https://www.uhfnyc.org/publications/881033

- http://www.bizjournals.com/albany/blog/health-care/2015/02/why-hospitals-are-spending-millions-of-dollars-on.html

Glossary Of Terms
The Makeup of Free Market Medicine: The National Picture Definitions and Distinctions

Note: Driven by both consumer demand and the prospect of new business and professional opportunities for physicians, "Membership Medicine" and "Convenient Care" have emerged over the past 15 years as free market healthcare delivery solutions. It's important to understand their definitions, services offered, roles in the healthcare economy and evolution.

The terminology and definitions below recognizes the impact of these new types of providers and the definitions speak to a the changing healthcare landscape, both politically, economically and socially. You will notice common goals of integrated care, patient-centered medical home solutions as well as overlap in services and how each may support primary care. There are primarily three healthcare sectors which makeup free market medicine:

- Membership Medicine

- Convenient Care

- Telemedicine

"Membership Medicine" is a collective term used to describe the subscription-based, healthcare delivery models for: Direct Primary Care (DPC); boutique; retainer-based medicine; and Concierge Medicine Models currently operating throughout the U.S. In Membership Medicine, the membership is available and affordable to many people, not just the wealthy. It may be in the form of a monthly payment option as many DPC Clinics offer or in a quarterly or annual retain payment, as most Concierge Medicine Doctors provider. It is a misconception that Physicians participating in this style of practice are solely doing so to experience more financial success.

"Convenient Care" is the collective term for urgent care centers and retail clinics—is a major development in the delivery of ambulatory care. Both retail clinics and urgent care centers offer walk-in services with extended evening and weekend hours, but important distinctions exist between the two models: Retail Clinics and Urgent Care Centers.

"Telemedicine" – Formally defined, telemedicine is the use of medical information exchanged from one site to another via electronic communications to improve a patient's clinical health status. Telemedicine includes a growing variety of applications and services using two-way video, email, smart phones, wireless tools and other forms of telecommunications technology. (Source: American Telemedicine Association)

Membership Medicine:
The National Picture Definitions and Distinctions

Boutique Medicine.

See definition for Membership Medicine.

Cash-Only Medicine.

See definition for Direct Primary Care (DPC).

Concierge Medicine.

Concierge medicine is a relationship between a patient and a primary care physician in which the patient pays an annual fee or retainer. This may or may not be in addition to other charges. In exchange for the retainer, doctors provide enhanced care. Concierge physicians care for fewer patients than in a conventional practice, ranging from 100 patients per doctor to 600-800, instead of the 3,000 to 5,000 that the average physician now sees every year.

All generally claim to be accessible via telephone or email at any time of day or night or offer some other service above and beyond the customary care provided. The annual fees vary widely, from US $10 per month to US $1,500 per year for an individual, with the lower annual fees being in addition to the usual fees for each service and the higher annual fees including most services.

Other terms in use include: boutique medicine; retainer-based medicine; and innovative medical practice design. The practice is also referred to as: membership medicine; concierge health care; private medicine; cash-only practice; direct care; direct primary care; DPC; and direct practice medicine.

While all concierge medicine practices share similarities, they vary widely in their structure, payment requirements, and form of operation. In particular, they differ in the level of service provided and the fee charged. At this writing, it has been estimated that concierge medicine and direct care physicians number approximately 12,000 physicians and/or physician clinics across the U.S.

"I suspect that employers will be the major reason for direct primary care membership/retainer-based practice growth in the coming years as they will essentially demand that level of service for their employees — and in so doing they will be reducing their company health care costs as a result of high quality primary care. The exact number of physicians in DPC practices is unclear but an estimate by Concierge Medicine Today in early 2014 pegs the known number at about 4,000 with about 8,000 others doing so but without fanfare [so in total, approximately 12,000]. More doctors will convert once the general population understands the advantages and begins to ask for it. There are many good reasons for an individual to connect with a direct primary care physician: better quality care, a return to relationship medicine and often a significant cost savings despite the fee." *-Dr. Stephen C. Schimpff is a quasi-retired internist, professor of medicine and public policy, former CEO of the University of Maryland Medical Center, senior advisor to Sage Growth Partners and is the author of The Future of Health-Care Delivery: Why It Must Change and How It Will Affect You*

Neil Chesanow of *Medscape* wrote in May 2014: According to the Association of American Medical Colleges, there were 817,850 active physicians in the United States in 2012, the latest year for which statistics are available.[2] How many of these doctors are in concierge or direct primary care practices? "We believe — and this is after years of verifying doctors, talking with actual doctors, talking with business leaders, and talking with physicians who are influencers — that there are slightly less than 4000 physicians who are verifiably, actively practicing concierge medicine or direct primary care across the United States, with probably another 8000 practicing under the radar," Michael Tetreault estimates. Matthew Priddy, whose organization includes physicians in both groups, figures that there are about 5000 concierge and direct primary care physicians nationwide. But he also believes that a sizable number of concierge and direct primary care physicians don't want to draw attention to themselves and keep a low profile. Right now, far more traditional doctors are telling surveyors that they plan to switch than actually appear to be doing it.

Direct Care Medicine.

See definition for Direct [Primary] Care.

Direct Care or Direct Primary Care (DPC).

Direct Primary Care (DPC) practices are distinguished from other retainer-based care models, such as concierge care, by lower retainer fees (82% cost less than $99/mo), which cover at least a portion of primary care services provided in the DPC practice; No insurance plan is involved, although patients may have separate insurance coverage for more costly medical services; Patients typically prefer to pay monthly vs. quarterly or annually; DPC patients typically come from the Generation X and Millennial population and earn a combined annual HH income of less than $100k.

DPC is primary and preventative care, urgent care, chronic disease management and wellness support through a monthly care fee, a patient (or an employer) pay to cover the specific primary care preventative care services. A DPC health care provider charges a patient a set monthly fee for all primary care services provided in the office, regardless of the number of visits. Because the insurance "middle man" is removed from the equation, all the overhead associated with claims, coding, claim refiling, write-offs, billing staff, and claims-centric EMR systems disappears.

DPC medical practices bypass insurance and go for a more 'direct' financial relationship with patients while also providing comprehensive care and preventive services for an affordable fee. DPC is a 'mass-market variant of concierge medicine, distinguished by its low prices.' Simply stated, the biggest difference between 'direct primary care' and retainer-based practices is that DPC takes a low, flat rate fee whereas concierge medicine models, (although plans may vary by practice) - usually charge an annual retainer fee and promise more 'access' to the doctor.

Direct primary care (DPC) is a term often linked to its companion in health care, 'concierge medicine.' Although the two terms are similar and belong to the same family, concierge medicine is a term that fully embraces or 'includes' many different health care delivery models, direct primary care being one of them.

Direct primary care practices offer a membership-based approach to routine and preventive care that can dramatically reduce health care costs for individuals, families and businesses.

At the core of a direct primary care facility is a medical practice dedicated to providing routine, everyday care, essential for the well-being and ongoing maintenance of a patient's health. This is where patients go for check-ups, vaccinations, sprained ankles, frequent headaches or other primary care services.

DPC Doctors know their patients. They have talked with their patients in detail, gotten to know them, treated past conditions and know what recurring problems are experienced. If a patient has a chronic illness, like arthritis or diabetes, their primary care provider is already a partner in management every step of the way. In the unlikely event of a life-threatening accident or disease, the Provider serves as the Patient's advocate, coordinating care across multiple providers, facilities, and prescriptions.

Source: DPCare.org

DPC and Membership Medicine:

As of late 2014, The DPC Journal finds that key leadership in the Direct Primary Care (DPC) industry, interviews and reports received from the business, employer and investment community operating in the DPC marketplace nationally, center around the number that there are more than 900+ DPC physicians ... and growing and growing at a rate of about 5-10% nationwide.

- DPC is primary and preventative care, urgent care, chronic disease management and wellness support through a monthly care fee, a patient (or an employer) pay to cover the specific primary care preventative care services.
- DPC practices are distinguished from other retainer-based care models, such as concierge care, by lower retainer fees, which cover at least a portion of primary care services provided in the DPC practice.
- Monthly fees at direct practices vary from $25-$85 per month or less. Patients prefer to pay monthly vs. quarterly or annually.
- DPC patients typically come from the Generation X and Millennial population and earn a combined annual HH income of less than $100k.

- A DPC health care provider charges a patient a set monthly fee for all primary care services provided in the office, regardless of the number of visits.
- No insurance plan is involved, although patients may have separate insurance coverage for more costly medical services.
- Since the insurance "middle man" is removed from the equation, all the overhead associated with claims, coding, claim refiling, write-offs, billing staff, and claims-centric EMR systems disappears.

Concierge Medicine/Boutique and Retainer-Based Care:

Throughout the past several years of surveying the market (2007-2015), discussing the question with numerous doctors, interviewing industry business leaders, private equity investors, business consultants, key industry physicians and membership medicine leadership nationally — *Concierge Medicine Today* finds that there are slightly less than 4,000 actively practicing Concierge Medicine physicians across the United States, with another 8,000 practicing in some form or model of "Membership Medicine" under the radar.

Dr. Thomas W. LaGrelius, MD said in an interview with *Daily Breeze*, a publication in the Los Angeles, CA area that "While it is true, as the AP reported, that more and more patients are joining our practices nationwide, the number of patients is not just in the thousands already but in the millions. While it is true that concierge practice is exponentially on the rise, the current number of such doctors is not just in the hundreds but in the thousands, perhaps tens of thousands. Most are below the radar. They work quietly and are never counted by bureaucrats."

- Annual fees at direct practices vary from $101-$225 per year. Patients pay annually vs. monthly.
- Concierge Medicine patients skew upper middle class, with typical household earnings between $125,000 and $250,000 a year. They also tend to be Baby Boomers, generally in their 50s to 80s, according to doctors interviewed.
- A greater breadth of primary care services covered by an annual retainer contract fee structure.
- Many Concierge Doctors also bill insurance or Medicare for actual medical visits, as the monthly "access fee" is only for "non-covered" services. This results in two subscriptions paid by patients — the concierge medicine fee, and the insurance premium. Importantly, a few concierge practices do not bill insurance for medical visits, as the monthly fees cover both access and primary care visits.

In a recent interview with *The Atlanta Journal Constitution* and *CNN Money*, a *Concierge Medicine Today* spokesperson said "We estimate that there are approximately 12,000 Doctors/Clinics Operating In "Membership Medicine" in The U.S. in 2015. This represents approx. 1% of All Licensed Physicians In The U.S. in 2014 or 5+% of all Licensed Primary Care Physicians In The U.S. in 2014."

Retainer-Based Medicine.

See definition for Membership Medicine.

Subscription-Based Medicine.

See definition for Membership Medicine.

Convenient Care:
The National Picture Definitions and Distinctions

Retail Medicine.

Retail clinics generally offer limited services for specific minor acute conditions with clear clinical guidelines; some are expanding their scope to include management of chronic illness. Nationally, there are some 1,900 retail clinics, receiving more than 6 million visits annually. Most (70 percent) are owned by pharmacies or big-box retailers, and rely on lower-cost providers—nurse practitioners and physician assistants. Their client base is primarily young adults (ages 18-44) and people without a usual source of care (61 percent, versus the national average of 20 percent).

Urgent Care.

Urgent care centers treat patients with higher-acuity conditions, similar to those treated in primary care but with an emphasis on episodic illness and minor trauma; nearly all provide simple lab tests, and most offer basic x-ray services. Nationally, an estimated 9,000 urgent care centers receive some 160 million visits annually. Ownership is divided among physicians/physician groups (35 percent), corporations (30 percent), hospitals (25 percent), and non-physician individuals or franchisers (7 percent). Nearly all centers have at least one physician on staff, about three-quarters of them board-certified, most often in family medicine.

Potential Benefit and Risk.

Lower costs. A number of studies have found lower costs per episode of care at both retail clinics and urgent care centers, compared with physicians' offices and emergency departments, despite concerns about stimulating increased utilization or unnecessary or duplicative follow-up care elsewhere.

Telemedicine:
The National Picture Definitions and Distinctions

Starting out over forty years ago with demonstrations of hospitals extending care to patients in remote areas, the use of telemedicine has spread rapidly and is now becoming integrated into the ongoing operations of hospitals, specialty departments, home health agencies, private physician offices as well as consumer's homes and workplaces.

Telemedicine is not a separate medical specialty. Products and services related to telemedicine are often part of a larger investment by health care institutions in either information technology or the delivery of clinical care. Even in the reimbursement fee structure, there is usually no distinction made between services provided on site and those provided through telemedicine and often no separate coding required for billing of remote services. ATA has historically considered telemedicine and tele health to be interchangeable terms, encompassing a wide definition of remote healthcare. Patient consultations via video conferencing, transmission of still images, e-health including patient portals, remote monitoring of vital signs, continuing medical education, consumer-focused wireless applications and nursing call centers, among other applications, are all considered part of telemedicine and tele health.

While the term tele health is sometimes used to refer to a broader definition of remote healthcare that does not always involve clinical services, ATA uses the terms in the same way one would refer to medicine or health in the common vernacular. Telemedicine is closely allied with the term health information technology (HIT). However, HIT more commonly refers to electronic medical records and related information systems while telemedicine refers to the actual delivery of remote clinical services using technology.

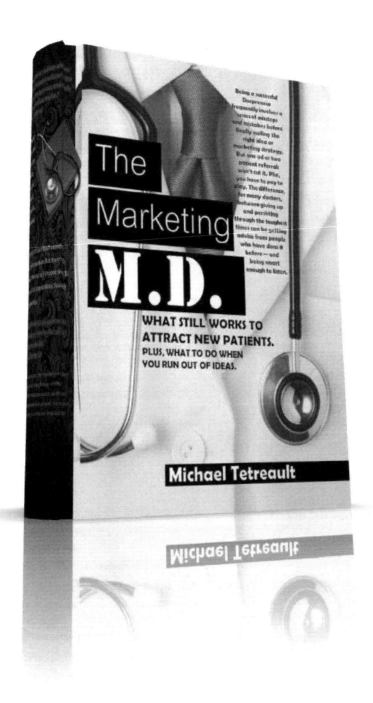

The Marketing M.D.

WHAT STILL WORKS TO ATTRACT NEW PATIENTS. PLUS, WHAT TO DO WHEN YOU RUN OUT OF IDEAS.

Michael Tetreault

Available At: www.DocPreneurPress.org

Appendices
Recommended Reading and Related Resources

Appendix 1 | Recommended Reading

Adding Refreshment Service In Your Concierge Practice
Available at: www.ConciergeMedicineToday.com

Appendix 2 | Recommended Reading

Many Malpractice Insurance Carriers Offer Discounts To Concierge/DPC Doctors Up To 45% Discount
Available at: www.ConciergeMedicineToday.com

Appendix 3 | Recommended Reading

Associations And Conferences Target Concierge And DPC Docs In 2014-2015
Available at: www.ConciergeMedicineToday.com

Acknowledgements

Disclaimer: While we make every effort to ensure that at the date of this book and its publication that the contact information below is up-to-date and accurate, we do recognize that the contact information, names, etc., are subject to change at any time. In addition to the resources, contacts, individuals and doctors mentioned in this book, we have provided you with a list of trusted physicians, resources, attorneys and businesses that you are welcome to reach out to at www.ConciergeMedicineToday.com or www.DirectPrimaryCare.com.

There are so many individuals, businesses and others who contributed to this body of work throughout the past few years. Without your proven expertise, dedication to your profession, enthusiasm for this book, and encouragement over the years, this resource would not be available. Here are some of the dedicated physicians, consultants and legal professionals who have made this book possible (Alphabetical Order):

Physician Contributors from
ARIZONA

Carrie Bordinko, MD
Consolaré Primary Care
Internal Medicine, CEO
4306 E. Desert Crest Drive
Paradise Valley, AZ 85253
Office: 602-350-2633
www.ConsolareMD.com

Eugene T. Conte, D.O., FAOCD
Cosmetic Dermatology Associates of
Prescott, AZ
212 S. Montezuma Street, Suite 6
Prescott, AZ 86303
Office: 928-515-2359
www.cosmeticdermatologyprescott.com

Susan Wilder, MD
LifeScape Premier
8757 East Bell Road
Scottsdale, AZ 85260
TEL: 480-860-5269
www.lifescapepremier.com

Physician Contributors from
COLORADO

Dr. David Tusek
Nextera Healthcare
4943 State HWY 52, Suite 240
Dacono, CO 80514
Office: 303-501-2600
www.nexterahealthcare.com

Dr. Clint Flanagan
Nextera Healthcare
4943 State HWY 52, Suite 240
Dacono, CO 80514
Office: 303-501-2600
www.nexterahealthcare.com

Note: Both Dr. Tusek and Dr. Flanagan and Nextera Healthcare can be found in multiple locations near the North Vista Medical Center, including: Longmont, CO; Firestone, CO; and Boulder, CO.

Physician Contributors from
CALIFORNIA

Shira Miller, MD
Integrative Center for Health & Wellness
13749 Riverside Drive, Suite 200
Sherman Oaks, CA 91423
Office: 818-574-8864
www.shiramillermd.com
www.facebook.com/menopausedoctor

Dr. Shira Miller
La Chiro Spa & Holistic Center
28047 Dorothy Drive #209
Agoura Hills, CA 91301
Office: 818-574-8864
www.shiramillermd.com

Dr. Lagrelius M.D., F.A.A.F.P.
Skypark Preferred Family Care
23451 Madison Street, Suite 140
Torrance, CA 90505
Office: 310-378-6208
www.skyparkpfc.com

M. Samir Qamar, MD
MedLion
851 South Rampart Blvd., Suite 110
Las Vegas, Nevada
Office: 855-696-3354
www.MedLion.com

Marcy Zwelling, MD
Choice Care
Private Medical Services
3771 Katella Avenue, Suite 108
Los Alamitos, California
TEL: 562-596-7584
www.z-doc.com

Physician Contributors from
CONNECTICUT

Sarah Mildred Gamble, D.O.
222 Railroad Avenue, Suite B
Greenwich, CT 06830
TEL: 203.869.2800
www.greenwichpuremedical.com

Physician Contributors from
FLORIDA

Jeffrey S. Gorodetsky, M.D.
Stuart, Florida Family Physician
433 East Ocean Boulevard
Stuart, FL 34994
Office: 772-223-4504
www.jeffreygorodetskymd.com
www.jsgmedicalpractice.com

Gary Price, MD, FACP
Concierge Physicians Southwest Florida
9722 Commerce Center Court
Fort Myers, FL 33908
Office: 239-415-1111
www.ConciergePhysiciansSWFL.com

Gary Price, MD, FACP – 2nd Location
Concierge Physicians Southwest Florida
2407 Periwinkle Way
Sanibel, Florida 33957
Office: 239-415-1111

Gary Price, MD, FACP – 3rd Location
Concierge Physicians Southwest Florida
24850 Burnt Pine Drive
Bonita Springs, Florida 34134
Office: 239-415-1111

Gary Price, MD, FACP – 4th Location
Concierge Physicians Southwest Florida
111 Ponce De Leon
Clewiston, Florida 33440
Office: 239-415-1111

Physician Contributors from
FLORIDA (Con't)

Stacey J. Robinson, MD
200 Central Avenue, Suite 280
St. Petersburg, FL 33701
TEL: 727-329-8859
www.RobinsonMed.com

Dr. Tiffany Sizemore-Ruiz, D.O.
Choice Physicians of South Florida
1409 SE 1st Ave
Fort Lauderdale, FL 33316
Office: 954-523-4141
www.ChoicePhysiciansSFL.com

Brian Thornburg, MSM, DO, PA, FAAP
Innovative Pediatrics
6017 Pine Ridge Road, Suite 148
Naples, FL 34119
Office: 239-348-3563 or
239-348-7337
www.InnovativePediatrics.com
www.ThornburgPediatrics.com

Physician Contributors from
GEORGIA

Dr. Caroline Abruzese
Personalized Healthcare, LLC
800 Mt. Vernon Hwy, NE Suite 160
Atlanta, GA 30328
Office: 404-303-8889
www.mypersonalizedhealthcare.com

Dr. Edward Espinosa
Buckhead Concierge Internal Medicine
91 W. Wieuca Road NE
Bldg. A Suite 1000
Atlanta GA 30342
Office :: 404-257-5585
www.bcimonline.com

Robert Lamberts, MD
General/Primary Care/Internist/Pediatrics
119 Davis Road, Suite 4-A
Augusta, GA 30907-0214
TEL: 706-504-9321
www.doctorlamberts.org

Dr. Robert Nelson
316 W. Main Street
Cumming, GA 30040
Phone: 470-297-8089
robertnelsonmd@encompasshd.com
www.encompasshd.com

Physician Contributors from
MARYLAND

Alexa Faraday, M.D.
Greater Baltimore Medical Center (GBMC)
6701 North Charles Street, Suite #4,106
Baltimore, MD 21204
Office: 855-372-5392
www.DrAlexaFaraday.com

Physician Contributors from
MICHIGAN

John August Blanchard, M.D.
6483 Citation Dr., Suite B
Clarkston, MI 48346
Office: 248-220-1560
www.PremierMD.com

John August Blanchard, M.D.
1627 W. Big Beaver Rd.
Troy, MI 48084
Office: 248.220.1560
www.PremierMD.com

Physician Contributors from
MISSOURI

Ann Riggs, DO
1306 C Platte Falls Rd
Platte City, MO 64079
TEL: 816-431-2150
http://www.directmedicalcare.net

Physician Contributors from
NEBRASKA

Joel Bessmer, MD, FACP
Members.MD
105 S. 90th Street
Omaha, NE 68114
Office: 402-779-8400
www.members.md

Physician Contributors from
NEW YORK

David Blende, D.D.S.
Specialty: Dentist, House Calls
150 East 58th Street
8th Floor Annex
New York, NY 10155
TEL: 646-461-1295
www.HouseCallDentists.com

Marina Gafanovich, MD
1550 York Avenue
New York, NY 10028
Office: 212-249-6218
www.mynycdoctor.com

Ronald Primas, MD
952 5th Avenue
New York, NY 10075
TEL: 212.737.1212
www.DrPrimas.com

Physician Contributors from
PENNSYLVANIA

Charles Whitney, M.D.
Revolutionary Health Services
1121 General Washington Memorial Blvd.
Washington Crossing, PA 18977
Office: 215-321-1371
www.RevolutionaryHealthServices.com

Physician Contributors from
TEXAS

Dr. Jennifer Chilek
Stone Creek Family Medicine
19782 Hwy 105 West, Suite 111
Montgomery, TX 77356
Office: 936-582-0220
www.stonecreekfamilymedicine.com

Chris Ewin, MD, FAAFP
One To One, MD, P.A.
5450 Clearfork Main St. Suite
460 Fort Worth, TX 76109
Office: 817-423-5121
www.121md.net

James Pinckney II, M.D.
Diamond Physicians
8222 Douglas Avenue, Suite 700
Dallas, TX 75225
Office: 214-395-3491
www.diamondphysicians.com

Physician Contributors from
UTAH

Michael Jennings, MD
4525 Wasatch Blvd. Ste 310
Salt Lake City, UT 84124
TEL:801-998-8492
www.PFPSLC.com

Physician Contributors from
VERMONT

Dr. David Bisbee, MD
53 Old Farm Road
Stowe, VT 05672
Office: 802-523-5020
www.davidbisbeemd.com

Alicia Cunningham, MD
Specialty: General/Primary Care/Internist
181 South Union St
Burlington, VT 05401
TEL: 802-881-9019
www.aliciacunningham.com

Physician Contributors from
WASHINGTON

Qliance (Corporate Office)
2101 Fourth Avenue, Suite 600
Seattle, WA 98121
Office: 877-754-2623

Garrison Bliss, MD
Qliance (Seattle Location)
509 Olive Way, Suite 1,607
Seattle, WA 98101-1721
Office: 206-913-4700
www.qliance.com

Erika Bliss, MD, FAAFP
Qliance (Seattle Location)
509 Olive Way, Suite 1,607
Seattle, WA 98101-1721
Office: 206-913-4700
www.qliance.com

Lawrence Greenblatt, D.O.
1407 116th Avenue NE, Suite 102
Bellevue, WA 98004
Office: 425-637-0636
www.cmadoc.com

Legal Analysts & Contributors
INCLUDE:

James (Jim) R. Taylor
Milligan Lawless, P.C.
5050 North 40th Street, Suite 200
Phoenix, Arizona 85018
Office: (602) 792-3503
Email: Jim@MilliganLawless.com
www.milliganlawless.com

Michael H. Cohen
Michael H. Cohen Law Group
468 North Camden Drive
Beverly Hills, California 90210
Office: 310.844.3173

Or

530 Lytton Ave, 2nd Floor
Palo Alto, California 94301
www.michaelhcohen.com

Jack Marquis
Smith Haughey Firm
170 College Avenue Suite 320
Holland, MI 49423
Office: (616) 723-8731
http://www.shrr.com/john-r-marquis

Industry Expertise Contributors to this work
INCLUDE:

The DocPreneur Institute
Physician Mentors & Coaching
Atlanta, GA
Office: (770) 455-1650
www.TheDocPreneur.org

Industry Consultants/Contributors
to this work INCLUDE:

Richard Doughty, *CEO*
Cypress Concierge Medicine
7984 Coley Davis Rd. Suite 101
Nashville, TN 37221
Office: (855) 493-7477
www.yourcypress.com

Specialdocs
660 LaSalle Place – Suite 202
Highland Park, IL 60035
Office: (847) 432-4502
www.Specialdocs.com

Nancy Latady
Latady Physician Strategies, LLC
Office: Phone: (781) 275-1415
Email: nlatady@latadyps.com
www.LatadyPhysicianStrategies.com

Bill Cossart
MedFirst Partners, LLC
President & CEO
Corporate Office:
Wayland, MA.
Office: (800) 939-1850
www.medfirstpartners.com

About The Authors

J. Catherine Sykes serves as the Publisher and Managing Director of *Concierge Medicine Today, The Direct Primary Care Journal* and other publications – which are online news agencies serving all sectors interested in this emerging healthcare industry. Ms. Sykes is a healthcare and marketing professional bringing over thirty years of experience in marketing, product and operations development, network development and management to clients and businesses which she serves.

Ms. Sykes has been responsible for development and implementation of numerous types of health care services products involving: medical/hospital; PHO; chiropractic; workers' compensation; dental; mental health; eldercare; Concierge Medicine and utilization management products and services. Her development efforts have been featured in the *Wall Street Journal, Business & Health, Employee Benefits News, Atlanta Business Chronicle, Business Atlanta, Managed Healthcare News, Bureau of National Affairs Reports, Chiropractic Economics, MCIC* and other prominent publications. Further experience includes: new market introduction of a large national HMO and numerous specialty provider networks; marketing responsibility for a major metropolitan business/medicine coalition to develop and market effective health care cost containment products/services under a Robert Wood Johnson Foundation Grant: Community Programs for Affordable Healthcare, and marketing and strategic planning responsibility for health care related marketing/advertising accounts. She has consulted with and served as an advisor to associations, corporations, non-profits, government advisory committees and other consultancies. Catherine has authored such titles as: *The Patient's Guide To Concierge Medicine; Why Choose Concierge Care* and more.

Ms. Sykes has been a featured speaker on health care issues at local, state and national forums. She was one of 15 managed care professionals invited by the American Chiropractic Association to participate in a national managed care summit to establish a Professional Responsibilities Matrix Work Group. She was honored in 2004 by the Business Advisory Council of the National Republican Committee as a Georgia Businessperson of the Year in Washington DC. She is a member of the National Association of Health Underwriters, the National Association of Female Executives, and has held positions on the Board of Directors for the Atlanta Health Underwriters Association, several managed care networks, in addition to a number of United Way agencies and Christian ministries.

Michael is a respected voice, Editor, community builder and industry authority in both Concierge Medicine and Direct Primary Care (DPC) delivery systems. Known especially for establishing the award winning and respected independent online news and trade publication platforms, The DPC Journal and Concierge Medicine Today. Michael is one of the world's leading Concierge Medicine and Membership Medicine spokespersons. He has authored such books as: *The Patient's Guide To Concierge Medicine*, *The DPC Consumer Guide*, *Branding Concierge Medicine* and *The Marketing MD*.

Michael is also a faculty member and Physician Mentor at The Docpreneur Institute (DPI) in Atlanta, GA, and serves as the Director of Marketing at Soteria Healthcare, an ancillary services managed care organization (MCO). As of late, Michael's latest books, *The Marketing MD*, *Branding Concierge Medicine* and *The 2015 Edition of The DPC Consumer Guide* have become best-selling Amazon Kindle titles and now rank regularly in the top 50 on Amazon.com e-books sold in the Medical Resources section.

His marketing and business development efforts have been featured in: *The Wall Street Journal*; *Town & Country Magazine*; *CNN Money*; *Huffington Post*; *NPR®*; *Marketplace®*; *TIME*; *Consumer Reports*; *SmartMoney*; *Heritage Foundation*; *The Boston Globe*; *LA Business Chronicle*; *Becker's Hospital Review*; *Outside Magazine*; *MarketWatch*; *Fox Business*; *Reuters*; and many others.

Among Mr. Tetreault's accomplishments is the creation of The Concierge Medicine Research Collective, a research data collection arm of CMT that partners with Universities, physicians, and legislators to survey a concierge physician population about various topics. Tetreault also developed private medicine's first mobile (App) application, "Concierge Doc", which features an online directory of concierge and direct care doctors, breaking industry news, a complete history of Concierge Medicine, definitions, a storefront and more -- available for free on Android's Marketplace Store and iTunes. Additionally, Tetreault has also developed two community health care and volunteer programs, *The Go Fish Project* and *Healthy Town USA*. *The Go Fish Project* is a benevolence program in which health care providers donate time, money and services to designated charities each year. *Healthy Town USA*, is an event management program that provides opportunity for health care professionals to volunteer and in turn connects them with world-class professional athletes. Under Mr. Tetreault's direction, these initiatives have developed marketing partnerships with: AARP; ADP; Dannon Yogurt; Habitat For Humanity; The United Way; Kaiser Permanente Health Plans; USAA Duathlon World and National Championships; ITU Duathlon World and National Championships; USA Triathlon; the Marine Corps Marathon and many others. Mr. Tetreault was the first public relations strategist to incorporate chiropractic health care services into the Marine Corps Marathon in 2003.

On a personal note, Michael serves as a business & fundraising consultant for many faith-based NPOs. He's a graduate of The Fund Raising School Program from the Center on Philanthropy at Indiana University Purdue University Indianapolis and graduated Cum Laude from Lee University in Tennessee where he received two Bachelor of Arts degrees, Marketing/Advertising and PR/Journalism. He is a recipient of the Inbound Marketing Certificate of Excellence by Inbound Marketing University (IMU), an award held by less than 2,000 individuals in the U.S.

A DOCTORS GUIDE TO CONCIERGE MEDICINE

First Edition.

Essential Startup Steps for Doctors Considering a Career in Concierge Medicine, DPC or Membership Medicine.

By Michael Tetreault and Catherine Sykes